Making Sense of Exercise Testing

Making Sense of Exercise Testing

Robert B. Schoene

Director, Internal Medicine Training Program
University of California San Diego School of Medicine
San Francisco, California

H. Thomas Robertson

Professor Emeritus, Medicine and Physiology and Biophysics
University of Washington
Seattle, Washington

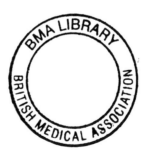

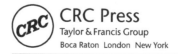

CRC Press

Taylor & Francis Group
Boca Raton London New York

CRC Press is an imprint of the
Taylor & Francis Group, an **informa** business

CRC Press
Taylor & Francis Group
6000 Broken Sound Parkway NW, Suite 300
Boca Raton, FL 33487-2742

© 2019 by Taylor & Francis Group, LLC
CRC Press is an imprint of Taylor & Francis Group, an Informa business

No claim to original U.S. Government works

Printed on acid-free paper

International Standard Book Number-13: 978-1-4987-7544-1 (Paperback)

Library of Congress Cataloging-in-Publication Data

Names: Schoene, Robert B., 1946- author. | Robertson, H. Thomas, author.
Title: Making sense of exercise testing / Robert B. Schoene, H. Thomas Robertson.
Other titles: Making sense (Boca Raton, Fla.)
Description: Boca Raton, FL : CRC Press/Taylor & Francis Group, 2018. |
Series: Making sense | Includes bibliographical references and index.
Identifiers: LCCN 2018006278| ISBN 9781498775441 (paperback : alk. paper) | ISBN 9780429470424 (ebook)
Subjects: | MESH: Exercise Test | Lung Diseases--diagnosis | Cardiovascular Diseases--diagnosis |
Exercise Tolerance
Classification: LCC RC685.C58 | NLM WG 141.5.F9 | DDC 616.1/0642--dc23
LC record available at https://lccn.loc.gov/2018006278

Visit the Taylor & Francis Web site at
http://www.taylorandfrancis.com

and the CRC Press Web site at
http://www.crcpress.com

Contents

Preface

In our shared 45 years as both clinical and scientific colleagues, we have sustained a fascination with all aspects of exercise physiology and pathophysiology. We believe that formal exercise testing provides essential insights into both the pathophysiology of exercise impairment from a wide range of disease conditions and the variations encountered in a wide range of athletes. We have devoted teaching time throughout our careers to introducing the concepts included in the interpretation of exercise testing to anyone willing to sit and listen to us.

This book reflects the perspectives we have accumulated in the conduct of our weekly exercise teaching conference at the University of Washington which is now in its 37th year. The primary focus of that conference has been to introduce trainees to the conduct and interpretation of the thousands of exercise tests that have been conducted at different laboratories at the University of Washington over those years. Our conference participants primarily include pulmonary, cardiology, and sports medicine fellows, with visits from nurses, technicians, coaches, and medical students and occasional guest presentations from local physicians, faculty, or visiting faculty. In writing this book, we hope to address a similarly diverse group of readers who would like to gain facility in the performance and interpretation of cardiopulmonary exercise tests, which should be an important part of the clinical evaluation of both patients and athletes of all sports.

There are several excellent comprehensive exercise books that have endured for multiple editions, and in addition, there are a number of brief monographs on exercise testing based primarily on pattern recognition. Our intent here is to establish a middle ground, first by limiting our discussion only to the events observed in the standard clinical progressive work exercise test (the cardiopulmonary exercise test or CPET), but also by including current information on the physiology and pathophysiology that underlie those responses. We believe that balance of test focus and physiologic mechanisms is most useful for clinicians who plan to undertake diagnostic testing. From roughly 1500 conferences with many hundreds of trainees and practitioners, we have gained insight into the more challenging exercise concepts that both experienced and neophyte clinicians may encounter, and we hope that this book will help readers along the fascinating pathway to attaining clinical exercise expertise.

Brownie and Tom

Authors

Dr. Robert B. Schoene is a graduate of Princeton University '68 and Columbia College of Physicians and Surgeons '72. He continued his training at the University of Washington School of Medicine in Internal Medicine and Pulmonary Medicine. He was on the faculty there from 1981–2003; his clinical and research endeavors were primarily critical care and exercise physiology, which led to his overseeing two of the exercise laboratories there. He also became involved in high-altitude research, which took him to Mt. Everest in 1981 to explore the limits of human performance, Denali in the mid-1980s to investigate high-altitude pulmonary edema, and the Andes over a couple of decades to investigate people living at high altitude. In 2003, he went to the UCSD School of Medicine to direct the Internal Medicine Training program and continue his work in pulmonary and exercise physiology. He presently is in the San Francisco Bay area practicing intensive care medicine as well as clinical exercise testing.

Dr. H. Thomas Robertson is a graduate of Colgate University '64 and Harvard Medical School '68. He completed his four-year medical residency at the University of Washington, interspersed by a two-year tour as a partially trained anesthesiologist with the United States Army. After a two-year pulmonary fellowship at the University of Washington, he joined the Pulmonary Division as a faculty member. Throughout his academic career, he divided his time roughly equally between teaching, care of hospitalized patients, and physiology research in pulmonary gas exchange. He is now an Emeritus Professor of Medicine and Physiology and Biophysics at the University of Washington. In retirement, he continues to exercise patients and conduct the weekly exercise conference at the University Hospital.

Introduction

This book is intended for clinicians who want to use the insights provided by exercise testing in the evaluation and care of patients with exercise-related symptoms. With that goal in mind, we have chosen to focus the material presented in this book on the progressive work exercise test, the universally applied clinical exercise testing protocol. The multiple measurements acquired in the course of a standardized cardiopulmonary exercise test (CPET) provide unique insight into the integrated function of the cardiovascular, respiratory, and muscular systems as a subject progresses from rest to a symptom-limited maximal exercise effort. While a number of simple office-based exercise protocols, such as stair-stepping or walk tests, have value in assessing overall impairment, those tests provide no diagnostic information. The information gained from a CPET can identify the exercise-limiting organ system and provide more specific information as to the pathophysiologic characteristics of that limitation. In addition to providing diagnostic information on patients with unexplained exercise limitation, a CPET is also used to characterize risk profiles for patients with heart failure, adult congenital heart disease, or pulmonary hypertension, and the test can provide diagnostic insight into performance impairment in athletes whose sport requires a sustained heavy exercise effort.

A symptom-limited maximal exercise test ends when a subject is no longer able to sustain that demand for increasing muscular effort. That effort failure during a CPET is ordinarily attributable to a limitation of maximal oxygen delivery to the exercising muscles which is the function of the cardiovascular system. However, maximal uptake of oxygen by the respiratory system and maximal utilization of the delivered oxygen to produce contractile power within the working muscles are also potential limiting factors in different disease conditions. Maximal exercise performance is dependent on all three systems, and exercise impairment in disease can arise from any combination of those three components (Figure 1.1).

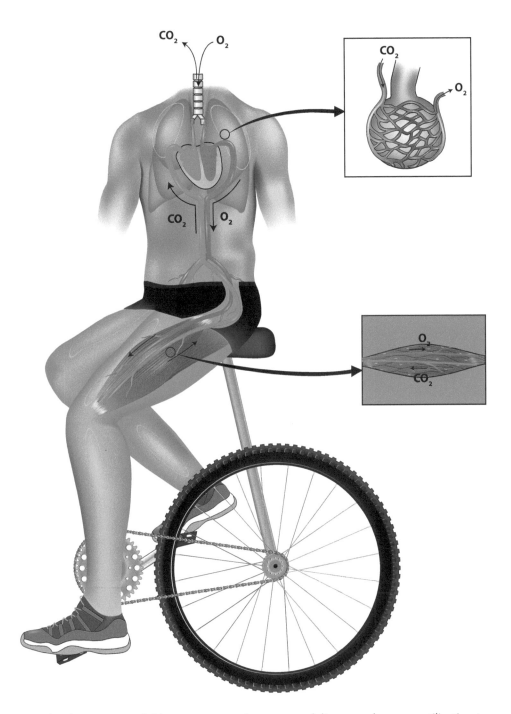

Figure 1.1 The three systems linking oxygen uptake, oxygen delivery, and oxygen utilization to muscle work.

Orientation to the cardiopulmonary exercise test

A standard clinical cardiopulmonary exercise test (CPET) acquires continuous measurements of metabolic, cardiovascular, and respiratory parameters over the course of an 8–15 minute effort in which exercise progresses incrementally from minimal movement to a maximal symptom-limited effort. This chapter first describes the equipment needed for these exercise measurements and then discusses the progressive work protocol that is used for all of these clinical studies.

EQUIPMENT REQUIRED FOR A CPET

The integrated commercial systems used for CPET studies incorporate input from several devices, but the measurements made on exhaled breath during exercise are the defining characteristics of a CPET study. Both the volume of exhaled breath and the concentrations of oxygen and carbon dioxide within that exhaled gas are monitored continuously, so the subject must exercise while breathing through a mouthpiece or mask connected to the measurement system. For systems that perform breath-by-breath measurements of both ventilation and gas exchange, any of several devices incorporated in the exercise mask or mouthpiece can monitor the flow rates within each exhaled breath. In addition, a sampling port for measurements of exhaled oxygen and carbon dioxide concentrations is located in that mask or mouthpiece assembly. The sampling rates for both gas flow and respiratory gas concentration measurements are high enough to permit accurate calculation of breath volume, oxygen uptake, and carbon dioxide output within each exhaled breath. For the simpler systems that do not provide breath-by-breath analysis, the patient's exhaled gas is directed through a mixing box, where volume measurement and respiratory gas concentrations are measured at the distal end of the mixing box. Both types of measurement systems are adequate for the majority of clinical applications, although the breath-by-breath systems can provide additional information on breathing patterns seen in some disease conditions.

In addition to the respiratory gas measurements, integrated CPET systems provide for continuous recording of standard 12-lead ECG for documentation of rate, rhythm, and ST changes during and after exercise. These systems usually can accept input from an automated blood pressure cuff and from a pulse oximeter. Alternately, manual blood pressure and pulse oximeter measurements can be recorded throughout exercise and recovery (Figure 2.1).

THE PROGRESSIVE WORK PROTOCOL

The progressive work protocol used for clinical studies has two characteristics that establish it as a diagnostic tool. First, a standard CPET utilizes an exercise mode that incorporates at least 50% of a subject's muscle mass, a criterion that is most conveniently met by exercise performed on either a cycle ergometer or a treadmill. Second, the progressive work protocol utilizing either ergometer or treadmill should last 8–15 minutes, starting from lowest-level exertion and progressing to a symptom-limited maximal effort.

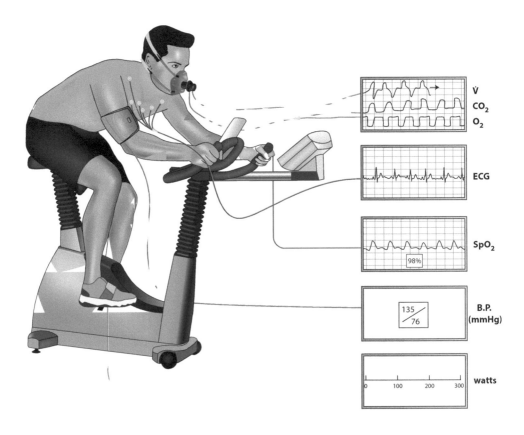

Figure 2.1 Subject on a cycle ergometer outfitted for a CPET, with device for airflow measurement and gas sampling leads attached to mask. Airflow and gas sampling leads are connected to system analysis equipment and computer, along with inputs from ECG, oximeter, blood pressure measurements and ergometer.

For either ergometer or treadmill exercise, the rate of increase of progressive exercise stress needs to be adjusted to allow the exercise subject to acquire 8–15 minutes of exercise data. For subjects exercised on a cycle ergometer, the progressive increments in cycling resistance are expressed in terms of watts of power generated. The exercise system setting that determines the rate of watt increase per minute must be adjusted according to subject size, as larger subjects can achieve larger absolute power outputs. To complete a 8–15 minute maximal exercise test, the chosen ergometer power increments must take into account both the subject's size and some estimate of the subject's maximal exercise capacity. For example, small elderly women might work at increments of 10 watts per minute and still be unable to last more than 8 minutes, while a large young male might last over 15 minutes utilizing increments of 25 watts per minute. For treadmill exercise, a standard protocol of increasing speed and grade ordinarily suffices, as subjects exercising on a treadmill are carrying their own body weight, exposing both small and large subjects to size-comparable exercise demands. However the increments of treadmill speed and grade still may need to be adjusted for estimated exercise capacity to achieve an 8–15 minute test that ends in a symptom-limited maximal exercise effort. Commercial exercise testing systems can automatically run previously selected progressions of ergometer or treadmill work rates during the test.

PRESENTATION OF THE MEASUREMENTS ACQUIRED IN A CPET

The software in integrated exercise systems uses the exercise measurements of gas flow and gas concentrations to calculate breath-by-breath measurements of tidal volume, oxygen uptake, and carbon dioxide output.

Exercise system software ordinarily presents the CPET data acquired throughout a test in a table of 20-second averaged blocks, including oxygen uptake, carbon dioxide output, tidal volume, minute ventilation, respiratory rate, heart rate, end-tidal oxygen, end-tidal carbon dioxide, ECG tracings, blood pressure, oxygen saturation, and power output for ergometer studies or treadmill time for treadmill studies. Ratios useful in test interpretation are calculated from these basic measurements. They include the respiratory "R" ($\dot{V}CO_2/\dot{V}O_2$), oxygen pulse ($\dot{V}O_2$/heart rate), and ventilatory equivalents for oxygen ($\dot{V}E/\dot{V}O_2$) and carbon dioxide ($\dot{V}E/\dot{V}CO_2$). The utility of all these measurements and ratios for test interpretation will be discussed in the following three chapters.

Breath-by-breath plots of oxygen uptake and carbon dioxide output during a progressive work test show substantial variability, but this variability is primarily attributable to the variability of breath size and does not represent measurement error or variability in muscle metabolism. As this

variability of measurements made at the mouth do not represent variability of the metabolic changes in the exercising muscle, the respiratory gas exchange measurements are ordinarily summed in 20-second bins and described in units of milliliter per minute.

POWER OUTPUT AND OXYGEN UPTAKE

Throughout a progressive work test, there is a consistent linear relationship between the oxygen consumption of the exercising subject and the power output achieved. For subjects being exercised on a cycle ergometer with appropriately chosen watt increments, every additional watt of power output is associated with a 10 mL/minute increase in oxygen consumption (Figure 2.2). For treadmill protocols that use a constant walking speed with progressive increases in treadmill grade, the relationship is linear. (Treadmill protocols that incorporate both incremental grade and incremental treadmill speeds also show a linear increase in oxygen consumption, with the exception that the walk-run transition produces a one-time bump in oxygen consumption.)

The measurement of oxygen consumption achieved in the final interval of a symptom-limited maximal effort represents a clinically accepted definition of maximal oxygen uptake ($\dot{V}O_2$ max). Some sources refer to this measurement as $\dot{V}O_2$ peak unless there is documentation of a sustained,

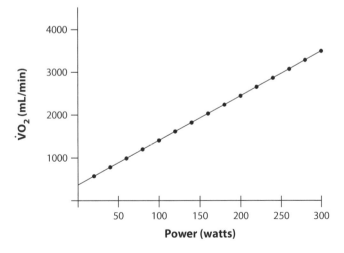

Figure 2.2 Graph of oxygen consumption versus watts of power expended during a CPET with subject exercised at 20 watt/minute increments and oxygen consumption averaged in 20-second bins.

unchanged oxygen consumption in the face of a continued increase in power output. We will use the term $\dot{V}O_2$ max for any symptom-limited effort. Using this less stringent definition, the $\dot{V}O_2$ max is still an exceptionally reproducible measurement, with a day-to-day variability for all subjects of no more that 2%–3%.

The physiologic events taking place during a CPET involve progressive adaptations of the exercising muscle groups, the circulatory system, and the respiratory system to keep pace with the increasing exercise intensity. The following three chapters will review the normal progression of exercise responses for each of those three linked organ systems as a subject progresses from the exercise warmup to a maximal exercise effort. The subsequent chapters will focus on system responses in different categories of disease, all from the perspective of observations made during a progressive work protocol.

3

Exercising muscle during a progressive work test

Leg fatigue is the most common limiting symptom that normal subjects describe at the end of a progressive work test. That transient failure of the exercising muscles could be attributed to any of several potential sources, but the choice of exercise mode and progressive work protocol of a standard clinical CPET make oxygen delivery to the exercising muscles the primary exercise-limiting factor. This chapter describes why the maximal effort expended during a CPET is primarily determined by the blood flow delivered to the exercising muscles. This chapter also describes the metabolic changes that take place within exercising muscles in the course of a progressive work test and how these changes influence the respiratory and cardiovascular responses observed in the course of a clinical exercise test.

- Exercise limitation during a work test
- Fuel utilization during a test
- ATP production during a test
- Lactate and acidosis during a test
- Muscular work efficiency and heat production

THE PRIMARY LIMITATION FOR EXERCISING MUSCLE DURING A PROGRESSIVE WORK TEST

The inability to sustain power output at the end of an exercise test could be attributed to any of the multiple steps involved in sustaining muscle work, including the events driving the cycle of muscle fiber contraction and relaxation, the maximal possible production capacity of adenosine triphosphate (ATP) within the muscle mitochondria, or

the maximal possible delivery of oxygen or carbon fuel sources to the mitochondria (Figure 3.1).

The use of either cycle ergometer or treadmill exercise for a maximal exercise test establishes the mechanism responsible for the exercising muscle failure at the end of a CPET. Both of those exercise modes require recruitment of more than 50% of the total muscle mass at maximal exercise effort. A maximal sustained exercise effort for any muscle group leads to dramatic vasodilation in the exercising muscle bed. However, if maximal vasodilation were allowed for more than 50% of the total muscle mass recruited during a standard CPET, the maximal cardiac output could not adequately support systolic blood pressure, leading to insufficient cerebral and coronary perfusion. Hence, during heavy exercise performed on either an ergometer or a treadmill, autonomic reflexes suppress the maximal possible vasodilation of arteries serving the exercising muscles, thereby protecting systolic pressure, but limiting maximal performance of those muscles. Hence, the maximal muscle performance attained during a CPET is limited by the fraction of the maximal cardiac output that can be allocated to the exercising muscles.

The influence of the total exercising muscle mass on maximal muscle blood flow has been demonstrated in exercise studies in which the subjects had catheters and flow sensors placed in one femoral vein, so that individual leg blood flow and leg oxygen consumption could be measured during cycle ergometer exercise (Figure 3.2). During a standard cycle ergometer progressive work test, measurements of maximal blood flow and leg oxygen consumption were acquired on the catheterized leg.

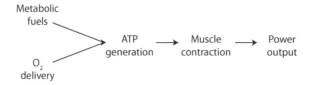

Figure 3.1 Possible sources of muscle contractile failure during a maximal effort in a CPET.

The subjects then re-exercised with only the catheterized leg pedaling the ergometer. The single-leg exercise measurements showed a 15% higher blood flow, oxygen consumption, and power output in the catheterized leg in comparison to the measurements made on the leg during the two-leg effort, documenting the influence of autonomic reflexes on the allowed muscle blood flow at maximal effort.

While the autonomic vascular response limiting maximal blood flow to exercising muscle during a maximal sustained effort poses one limitation to maximal expended effort, that observation does not rule out the other potential mechanisms for muscle failure with maximal effort that were considered above. However, the primacy of maximal oxygen delivery to muscle as the predominant progressive work test limitation has been demonstrated by experiments that increase the oxygen content of arterial blood. A subject exercised while breathing 100% oxygen will have a 10% increase in arterial oxygen content compared with exercise while breathing room air. While this intervention increases maximal exercise capacity and maximal oxygen uptake, the net increase achieved is only about 3% rather than 10%. Likewise, an erythrocyte transfusion to increase the hemoglobin concentration by 10% will increase the measured maximal oxygen uptake, but again by only 4% or 5%. The failure of these interventions that increase oxygen delivery to produce a strictly proportional increase in oxygen consumption suggests the existence of other limitations to maximal muscle oxygen uptake. The most important of those factors is likely the presence of an oxygen diffusion limitation between muscle capillary lumen and muscle mitochondria. Nevertheless, experiments described above illustrate that any intervention that increases oxygen content delivered to exercising muscle during a CPET will increase maximal exercise capacity and maximal oxygen uptake.

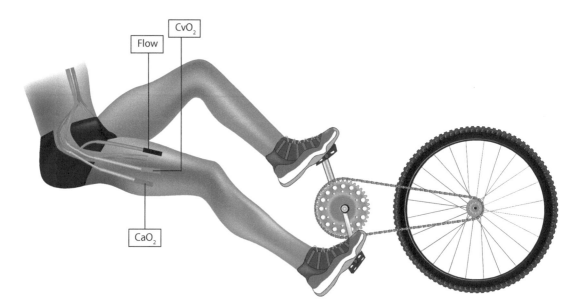

Figure 3.2 Subject exercising with femoral catheters placed for measurements of leg arterial and venous blood oxygen content, and venous blood flow in one leg.

If a progressive work protocol is applied to a smaller fraction of total muscle mass (such as that described in the single exercising leg study), the maximal sustained power attained in that setting is more representative of the strength of the exercising muscles. For example, a more specific test of cycling power, the Wingate test, measures the highest power output a subject can sustain on a cycle ergometer during a 30-second maximal effort. For such very short duration tests, the maximal power generated is not dependent on oxygen delivery. However using the standard clinical treadmill or ergometer protocols, by virtue of both test duration and involvement of a large fractional mass of muscle, the maximal power output attained in those protocols is primarily dependent on the maximal possible cardiac output delivered to the exercising muscles rather than muscle strength.

THE UTILIZATION OF FUELS DURING A PROGRESSIVE WORK TEST

The generation of ATP requires carbohydrate and fatty acid fuel sources in addition to oxygen supply. Muscle cells contain stores of both glycogen and lipid, and those local fuels are the primary metabolic resources utilized during the relatively short duration of a CPET, with lesser contributions from blood-borne glucose and triglycerides. The proportional use of carbohydrate or fat by exercising muscle depends on the level of effort required. The respiratory quotient (RQ), the ratio between CO_2 production ($\dot{V}CO_2$) and oxygen consumption ($\dot{V}O_2$), reflects the balance between fat and carbohydrate metabolism. A fasting subject at rest will primarily metabolize fat, with a corresponding RQ value as low as 0.70, whereas the same subject given a large ingested glucose load will have an RQ over 0.90. During an exercise test, the $\dot{V}CO_2/\dot{V}O_2$ ratio (termed the respiratory R rather than RQ because it is not a steady-state measurement) is measured continuously and reflects that effort-dependent changing pattern of fuel utilization. For a fasting subject, fat serves as the primary fuel source during the initial stages of exercise, giving R measurements less than 0.8 in fasting subjects, but as exercise intensity increases, there is progressively more dependence on carbohydrate utilization, producing an increase in the respiratory R value (Figure 3.3).

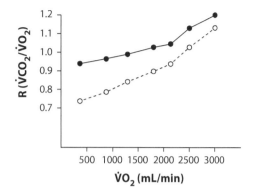

Figure 3.3 Increases in the respiratory R value during exercise for a fasting subject (open circles) and the same subject after consuming a high-carbohydrate meal (closed circles).

While the metabolism-dependent RQ cannot exceed 1.0, during an exercise test the respiratory R will exceed 1.0 with the onset of the normal metabolic acidosis of heavy exercise and its associated compensatory increase in ventilation. The additional CO_2 in the exhaled breath during short-duration heavy exercise reflects the tissue bicarbonate buffering of the exercise acidosis and a washout of CO_2 stores from systemic tissues, in addition to the metabolically generated CO_2. Hence, the progressively increasing respiratory R value during heavy exercise reflects both changes in the proportional fuel utilization and the increased stimulation to ventilation in response to the progressive metabolic acidosis of heavy exercise.

The fallacy of a "fat burning zone"

Many commercial gym exercise devices describe lower levels of sustained work as "fat burning zones," with the implication that, at higher levels of exertion, fat is no longer utilized as a fuel. That incorrect assumption arose from a misinterpretation of an old illustration that showed carbohydrates were a progressively more important source of fuel as the level of exertion increased. That is certainly true, but even though the contribution of fat metabolism is relatively lower during intense exertion, the absolute quantity of fat utilized by exercising muscle (or "burned") continues to increase with the level of exertion.

ATP GENERATION WITHIN MUSCLE DURING EXERCISE: THE SHORT VERSION

Muscle-bound ATP provides the energy for each muscle contraction, with a subsequent release of ADP (adenosine diphosphate), phosphate, and a hydrogen ion. These contraction byproducts readily diffuse back into the mitochondria within the muscle cell, where ATP is regenerated. The rate of ATP generation appears to be dependent on the concentration of ADP as the cellular concentration of ADP increases during sustained muscle activity (Figure 3.4).

The generation of ATP takes place in two different locations within the muscle cell: one site that is oxygen independent and one that is oxygen dependent. Within the cell cytosol, ATP is synthesized from ADP during the breakdown of glucose or glycogen in the process of glycolysis. That series of reactions produces two molecules of the three-carbon compound pyruvate, two free-hydrogen ions, and two molecules of ATP per glucose molecule. That process is not dependent on the presence of oxygen. However, the most important ATP generation site is within the mitochondria, where both the pyruvate generated in the cytosol from glucose or glycogen and free fatty acids are taken up to serve as the fuel sources for the multiple steps needed to initiate oxidative phosphorylation. The energy harvested from that sequence of mitochondrial oxygen-dependent reactions is used to synthesize ATP. The complete oxidation of one molecule of glucose via the mitochondrial respiratory chain will provide energy for the synthesis of up to 30 molecules of ATP. Glycolysis alone generates only two ATP molecules per glucose, and if the glycolytic production of pyruvate exceeds the mitochondrial uptake of pyruvate, the excess pyruvate is converted to lactate ion (Figure 3.5).

As the exercise work load progresses, the capacity of mitochondria to utilize free fatty acids is limited, and carbohydrate becomes a progressively more important mitochondrial fuel source. This shift is illustrated by the increasing values of R during a CPET, as illustrated in Figure 3.3. At heavier levels of exertion, muscle sympathetic nerves release more norepinephrine, further stimulating glycolysis from muscle glycogen stores. This metabolic pathway produces three ATP, two NADH, two pyruvate, and two H^+ for every molecule of muscle glycogen utilized. Eventually more pyruvate is produced than the mitochondria can utilize, and the excess pyruvate left in the cytosol combines with the NADH to produce NAD^+ and a lactate anion. While accelerated glycolysis during heavy exercise provides an additional source of ATP, it comes with the cost of producing a progressive metabolic acidosis that also contributes to exercise-limiting symptoms. Hence, during heavy non-sustainable exercise, lactate accumulates in proportion to the intensity of the glycolysis, but it is the process of glycolysis that generates the free hydrogen ions, not the lactate anion. Practically speaking, however, the onset of rising arterial lactate levels is a reliable marker for the onset of the metabolic acidosis that characterizes heavy non-sustainable exercise (Figure 3.8).

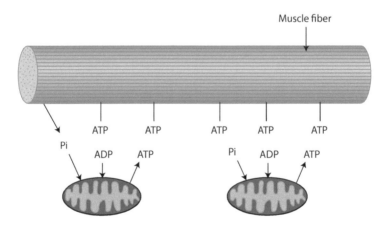

Figure 3.4 Mitochondria within muscle fibers generate most of the ATP needed for contraction, using the ADP and inorganic phosphate that were byproducts of previous muscle contraction.

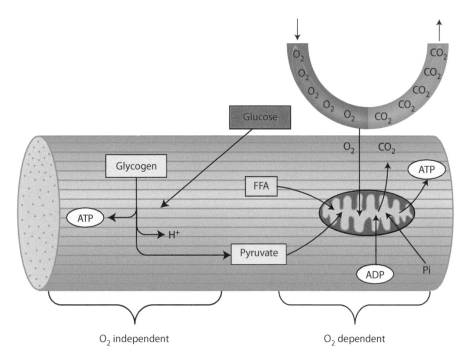

Figure 3.5 The oxygen-independent and oxygen-dependent utilization of carbon fuels to regenerate ATP within the working muscle cell.

Additional detail on the mitochondrial generation of ATP

Three different chemical processes take place within the mitochondria that lead to the oxidation of pyruvate and fatty acid to CO_2 and water and add the high-energy phosphate to ADP to regenerate ATP. First, the pyruvate and free fatty acids are drawn in to the mitochondrial cytosol, where they are both processed to a two-carbon acetyl group linked to coenzyme A. The acetylCoA then contributes the acetyl group into the citric acid (or Krebs) cycle. Each complete cycle of this reaction chain strips off electrons and hydrogen atoms, producing three NAD^+ to NADH reductions and one FAD to $FADH_2$ reduction, which constitute the energy sources for the next process. In addition, with each cycle, two carbons are expelled as CO_2 (Figure 3.6).

The next chemical process requires the double membrane structure of the mitochondrion, the inner membrane of which contains the complex of respiratory chain molecules. The NADH (and $FADH_2$) molecules derived from the citric acid cycle pass electrons and hydrogen ions into this chain, and the energy released from that oxidation of NADH pumps hydrogen ions into the space between the inner and outer mitochondrial membranes, creating a high chemical energy gradient across the inner membrane. The final enzyme of the respiratory chain is cytochrome oxidase, which combines four electrons that were passed along the respiratory chain with two oxygen molecules and four H^+ ions to produce two molecules of H_2O. As long as there is available oxygen to draw electrons across the respiratory enzyme chain and available NADH, those enzymes continue to build the hydrogen-ion concentration gradient between the inner and outer mitochondrial membranes. The respiratory chain remains fully functional even at the very low partial pressures of oxygen seen in maximally working muscle (Figure 3.7).

The final step leading to ATP regeneration from ADP requires the enzyme ATP synthetase, which is located on the inner mitochondrial membrane. The enzyme uses the energy

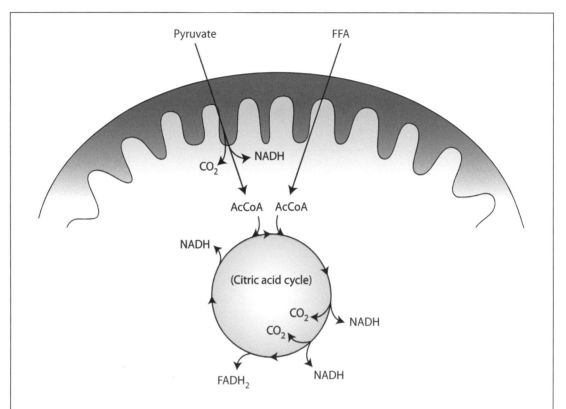

Figure 3.6 Pyruvate and FFA enter the mitochondria, are converted to acetylCoA, and enter the citric acid cycle. Each turn of the cycle spins off two CO_2 molecules and generates high-energy NADH and $FADH_2$ from NAD^+ and FAD.

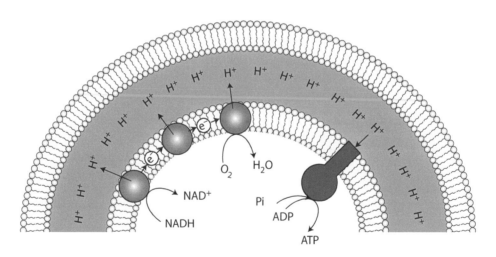

Figure 3.7 The respiratory chain molecules on the inner mitochondrial membrane accept electrons (e^-) from NADH and pump H^+ ions into the inter-membrane space. In the final respiratory chain step, oxygen reacts with electrons and H^+ to produce water. The accumulated energy from the elevated H^+ concentration within the paired membranes drives ATP synthetase, making ATP from ADP and inorganic phosphate (Pi).

from the hydrogen-ion gradient between the membranes to add the high-energy phosphate group to ADP, creating ATP.

The efficacy of ATP production is dependent not only on adequate oxygen and NADH supply, but also on an intact inner mitochondrial membrane to sustain the high H$^+$ ion concentration difference. If hydrogen ions can leak back across that inner membrane, oxygen consumption will continue, but less ATP will be produced. It appears that a "leaky" inner mitochondrial membrane will develop with aging and possibly also with some disease processes. The exercise effect of a leaky inner mitochondrial membrane is that a higher oxygen consumption will be needed to accomplish a given work rate.

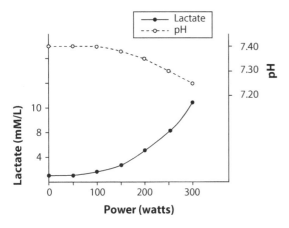

Figure 3.8 Measurements of arterial pH and lactate acquired at 2-minute intervals during a CPET.

During non-sustainable heavy exercise, the pH within working muscle will drop from a resting value of 7.0 to as low as 6.3, a result of both the hydrogen ions produced by maximal glycolysis and the increasing production of CO_2 at the highest possible levels of aerobic metabolism. The PO_2 of blood exiting the exercising muscles at maximal effort during a CPET will ordinarily be less than 25 mmHg, with values of 15 mmHg or less observed in well-trained athletes. The muscle hypoxemia, respiratory and metabolic acidosis, and hyperkalemia are all products of maximal muscle work, maximal mitochondrial function, and accelerated glycolysis at the end of a CPET effort.

LACTATE, ACIDOSIS, AND EXERCISE

The appearance of lactate in the blood in the later stages of a progressive exercise test was originally interpreted as a sign of exercise-limiting hypoxia in the muscles. There is now abundant evidence demonstrating that the original concept of exercise lactic acidosis as a consequence of muscle hypoxia is simply not correct. Mitochondria can continue to generate ATP at maximal rates at partial pressures of oxygen as low as 2–3 mmHg. Furthermore, lactate ion produced during exercise is the substrate of choice for myocardial metabolism and is also utilized by the non-maximally stressed skeletal muscles. Although the role of the liver in metabolizing lactate is still emphasized in many biochemistry textbooks, exercise-induced lactate is rapidly consumed by cardiac and skeletal muscle, with minimal liver participation during heavy exercise. The fast-twitch muscle fibers are the primary site for glycolysis and lactate production during a maximal effort. The proportion of fast-twitch fibers in muscle is determined both by the specific anatomic muscle group and the genetic makeup of the individual. For the muscles of locomotion involved during a CPET, there is substantial variability among normal individuals in the proportion of fast-twitch fibers within those muscles. Because of that variability among normal subjects in the proportion of fast-twitch fibers within muscle, there is a corresponding variability in lactate levels achieved with maximal effort. Hence, the level of arterial lactate observed immediately following a maximal effort is primarily determined by an individual's inherited proportion of glycogen-rich fast-twitch muscle, rather than the intensity of exercise effort attained.

Regardless of the historical confusion concerning the interpretation of exercise lactate levels, the appearance of lactate in the arterial blood reliably heralds the onset of the metabolic acidosis of normal heavy exercise and is a very useful marker in the clinical interpretation of a CPET. The onset of metabolic acidosis during exercise also represents the attainment of a level of exertion that the subject will not be able to sustain for more than a few minutes. The increasing arterial concentration of lactate anion and the associated metabolic acidosis also mark a point during a progressive work test associated with augmentation of exercise ventilation (the ventilatory or lactate threshold) and augmented increases in systolic blood pressure.

EXERCISE HEAT PRODUCTION AND THE EFFICIENCY OF MUSCULAR WORK

From an engineering perspective, muscular work is simply work performed by a chemical engine. Like any engine, muscle expends energy to perform work and also wastes the majority of that energy in the form of heat. Our exercising muscles are not particularly efficient. For example, if a subject pedaling on a cycle ergometer at 50 watts is then ramped up to an exercise load of 150 watts, the extra 100 watts of power generated will be associated with well over 200 additional watts of heat generation. While the 8–15 minute duration of a progressive work test is not sufficient to appreciably raise temperature for most subjects, elite-level athletes who can attain high power outputs may raise core temperatures by over 2°C during a standard duration test.

As oxygen consumption during exercise is directly related to fuel production (ATP) and muscle power output, a simple estimate of muscle efficiency can be made from the relationship between oxygen consumption and power output during

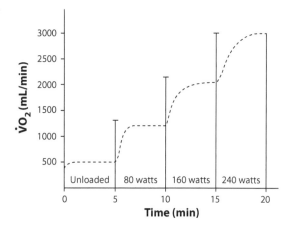

Figure 3.9 The time course of increases in oxygen consumption during four 5-minute exercise bouts at constant power output increments of 80 watts. Note that reaching a steady oxygen consumption takes longer with each higher power output, but that each 80-watt increment increases oxygen consumption by 800 mL/min (10 mL O_2/watt).

a steady-state exercise test performed on a cycle ergometer. For example, if a normal subject has oxygen consumption measured after pedaling an ergometer at 10 watts for several minutes, a repeat measurement after pedaling at 110 watts for several minutes will demonstrate an increase in oxygen consumption of 1000 mL. In short, comparing two different steady-state power outputs, there will be a very reproducible ~10 mL O_2 per watt difference in oxygen consumption (Figure 3.9).

SUMMARY POINTS

- Ergometer and treadmill exercise incorporate a large fraction of the total muscle mass, and this constraint necessitates some limitation of maximal blood flow to exercising muscle to permit adequate cerebral and coronary perfusion.
- Maximal oxygen consumption and maximal power output generated during a standard clinical CPET are primarily determined by the maximal

delivery of oxygenated blood to the exercising muscle.
- Muscle fuel utilization during a CPET utilizes muscle fatty acids at lower levels of exercise, with progressively greater contribution from muscle glycogen-derived carbohydrate at higher levels of exercise.
- The mitochondria within muscle cells can continue to produce increasing quantities of ATP during a progressive work protocol

until the delivery of oxygen-containing blood limits further increases in ATP production.

- With higher levels of exercise, muscle norepinephrine triggers glycolysis, and this process generates modest additional quantities of ATP and both hydrogen ions and lactate. During a CPET, the onset of this metabolic acidosis indicates a level of exercise that cannot be continued for a sustained period of time.

- During a progressive work test, the onset of the metabolic acidosis of heavy exercise is associated with a reproducible augmentation of exercise ventilation known as the ventilatory (or "anaerobic") threshold.

4

Cardiovascular system during a progressive work test

As described in the previous chapter, the maximal sustained exercise capacity of the working muscles during a CPET is primarily limited by the maximal capacity of the circulatory system to deliver oxygenated blood to the working muscles. The eight- to twelve-fold increase in oxygen consumption observed in normal subjects during a progressive work test requires both a substantial increase in cardiac output and redirection of most of that increased cardiac output to the exercising muscles. Although the blood flow to skeletal muscle only utilizes about 15% of the cardiac output at rest, there is a dramatic reallocation of flow during maximal exercise, so that up to 85% of the increased cardiac output is delivered to the exercising muscles. This chapter describes the following cardiovascular responses that take place to maximize that delivery:

- Factors determining oxygen delivery to muscle
- Exercise heart-rate response
- Exercise stroke-volume response
- The systemic reallocation of blood flow during exercise
- The O$_2$ pulse as a stroke-volume estimate
- Blood pressure response during exercise
- Delivery of oxygen within exercising muscle

THE FICK EQUATION TO DESCRIBE OXYGEN DELIVERY

The progressive increases in oxygen consumption during a cardiopulmonary exercise test require increases in heart rate, stroke volume, and more complete extraction of oxygen from arterial blood. Those cardiovascular responses to increase oxygen delivery during a progressive work test are concisely described by a rearrangement of the Fick equation. The original equation was employed to calculate cardiac output (the product of heart rate and stroke volume) by dividing measurements of oxygen consumption by the difference between arterial oxygen content and mixed venous oxygen content. A rearrangement of the terms in the Fick equation provides a useful tool to follow each of the factors that contribute to increasing oxygen delivery during a progressive exercise test (Figure 4.1).

During exercise, increases in both heart rate and stroke volume combine to increase the overall cardiac output. The increased oxygen extraction from mixed venous blood is achieved by direction of the majority of blood flow to the actively exercising muscles and reducing blood flow to other organ systems. During a standard CPET, we only have measurements of oxygen consumption, heart rate, and arterial oxygen saturation, but with those measurements, we can gain information about each of the three circulatory adaptations that increase oxygen delivery to muscle during a progressive work test.

EXERCISE HEART RATE

During a progressive work test, the heart rate increases in a nearly linear fashion throughout the test, in parallel with the increases in power required by ergometer settings or treadmill speed and grade (Figure 4.2).

$$\dot{V}O_2 = \left(\begin{array}{c} \text{Stroke} \\ \text{volume} \end{array} \right) \times \left(\begin{array}{c} \text{Heart} \\ \text{rate} \end{array} \right) \times \left(\begin{array}{cc} \text{Content} & \text{Content} \\ \text{arterial } O_2 & \text{venous } O_2 \end{array} \right)$$

Figure 4.1 Fick equation solved for oxygen consumption (in liters of oxygen per minute) as the product of heart rate (in beats per minute), stroke volume (in liters of blood), and the arterial-venous oxygen content difference (in liters of oxygen per liter of blood).

Some highly motivated subjects at maximal effort will demonstrate a plateau in the exercise heart rate despite increasing power demands, but this cannot be sustained for more than a minute or two and is not associated with any additional increase in oxygen consumption. The normal maximal exercise heart rate can be roughly estimated from the following relationship:

$$\text{Maximal HR} = 220 - \text{Age in years}$$

Better population estimates of maximal exercise heart rate include fits separated by sex (with female data somewhat less dependent on age compared to the above equation), but for interpretation of an individual test result, the more important insight is to understand that there is a large range of maximal exercise heart rates among normal subjects regardless of age or sex. For a 40-year-old subject, an estimated normal maximal heart rate would be 180 beats per minute, but with a standard deviation of 12 beats per minute. That is, 32% of the normal 40-year-old subjects would have maximal heart rates below 168 or above 192 beats per minute. There is no appreciable day-to-day variability in maximal exercise heart rate, so these differences represent true biologic variability among normal subjects.

Because of the range of normal variability in maximal exercise heart rate, maximal heart rate attained is not a reliable indicator of whether or not a subject gave a truly maximal effort. In addition, among healthy normal subjects, the maximal exercise heart rate attained is not appreciably linked with either the overall maximal oxygen uptake or the level of training. However, a larger range of increase in heart rate between rest and maximal effort is seen in subjects with high maximal oxygen uptakes. For example, a normal 30-year-old woman with a resting heart rate of 70 beats/min and a maximal rate of 190 beats/min would have an exercise heart rate range of 120 beats. In comparison, a 30-year-old, elite-level cyclist with the same maximal exercise heart rate of 190 beats/min but a resting rate of 40 beats/min would have a larger exercise heart rate range of 150 beats. As both women would have the same weight-corrected resting oxygen consumption, their heart rate range difference is simply a manifestation of the athlete's larger stroke volume that provides her a larger maximal cardiac output and oxygen delivery.

The choice of cycle ergometer or treadmill has a small influence on the maximal exercise heart rate attained. As a rough estimate, an average subject will reach a maximal exercise heart rate that is 4%–8% greater on a treadmill in comparison to a maximal effort on a cycle ergometer. This difference appears to be secondary to a higher fractional muscle mass required for a treadmill running and will also be associated with a higher maximal oxygen uptake on the treadmill. The maximal exercise heart rate difference between ergometer and treadmill exercise is most apparent with well-trained runners and is smallest with well-trained cyclists.

EXERCISE STROKE VOLUME

While stroke volume increases with upright exercise, the majority of that increase comes with the onset of exercise. Stroke volume is dependent on preload, and when a subject moves from supine to upright posture, blood pools in the dependent

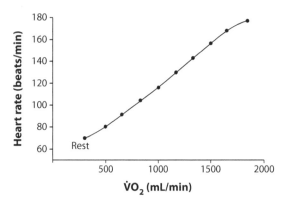

Figure 4.2 A typical CPET heart-rate response during a CPET.

leg veins, thereby reducing the stroke volume in comparison to measurements made in the supine posture. However, with the onset of upright exercise, the stroke volume increases back to its value in supine posture. This increase in stroke volume at the onset of exercise demonstrates the important role of the dependent veins in maintaining stroke volume during upright exercise. A unique human anatomic adaptation to upright posture is the presence of large venous plexuses surrounded by the calf muscles. During exercise the periodic contraction of the calf muscles surrounding the veins, in concert with functioning venous valves, creates a venous pump that augments the venous return to the thorax during upright exercise. In addition to the effective venous pump in the exercising legs, exercise initiates an increase in sympathetic tone that produces constriction of the capacitance veins and further augments the cardiac preload. Once these adaptations are initiated in moderate-level exercise, however, the stroke volume does not increase appreciably in normal subjects as the level of exertion increases to a maximal effort. Stroke volume will normally increase by about 30% with the initiation of moderate exercise in comparison with standing rest (Figure 4.3).

Normal resting stroke volume for subjects of the same size shows a substantial range of normal just as there was a range of normal with maximal exercise heart rate. Unlike heart rate, stroke volume is dependent on the size of the subject, but even when measured stroke volume is adjusted for body size (conventionally by dividing the measured stroke volume by estimated body surface area in square meters), there remains a large range of normal variability in stroke volume. Although the variability of normal maximal heart rate is not well correlated with maximal oxygen uptake, the variability of stroke volume among normal subjects accounts for a major part of the variability among individuals in maximal cardiac output.

ARTERIAL-VENOUS EXTRACTION AND THE REALLOCATION OF BLOOD FLOW DURING EXERCISE

At rest, the majority of the cardiac output is distributed to the heart, brain, splanchnic circulation, and kidneys, and the mixed venous oxygen saturation returning to the pulmonary artery is around 75%. With sustained maximal effort, the mixed venous saturation drops to 20% or 25%, and 85% of that increased cardiac output is directed to exercising muscle. The progressive decrease in the oxygen saturation of mixed venous blood (measured at the pulmonary artery) during a progressive work test is almost linearly related to the intensity of exercise effort. The mixed venous oxygen saturation during exercise reflects the mix between blood perfusing the exercising muscles (where oxygen extraction can exceed 90% at maximal effort) and the blood perfusing the rest of the body (Figure 4.4).

The mixed venous blood entering the pulmonary artery includes flow from all organ systems, but as the level of exertion increases, that flow is reduced in both the renal and splanchnic beds, a

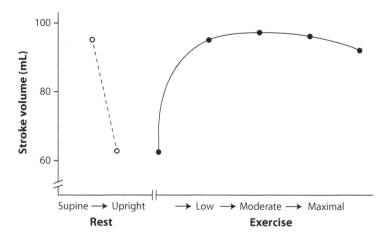

Figure 4.3 Changes in stroke volume between supine posture, upright standing, and during progressive upright exercise.

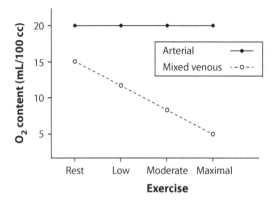

Figure 4.4 The nearly linear decrease in mixed venous oxygen content during a progressive work test, while arterial oxygen content remains unchanged.

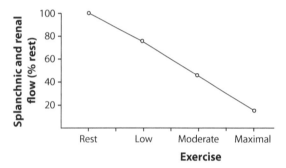

Figure 4.5 Progressive reduction in both splanchnic and renal blood flow with level of exertion, described as a percent of the resting values.

reduction that is in proportion to the level of effort expended. Coronary perfusion during exercise is enhanced by both the increased systolic pressure and intrinsic vasodilation, and central nervous system perfusion is unchanged (Figure 4.5).

THE O$_2$ PULSE MEASUREMENT

Of the three circulatory determinants of maximal oxygen uptake, (heart rate, stroke volume, and a-vO$_2$ difference) only heart rate is directly measured during a routine progressive exercise test. However given that normal stroke volume remains constant after the onset of exercise (Figure 4.3) and the very consistent relationship between the extent of a-vO$_2$ extraction and the level of effort expended (Figure 4.4), a useful measurement obtained from exercise test data is the O$_2$ pulse. The O$_2$ pulse

measurement is based on a rearrangement of the Fick equation, dividing the oxygen consumption by the heart rate:

$$\text{Fick equation}: \dot{V}O_2 = (\text{Heart rate})$$
$$\times (\text{Stroke volume})$$
$$\times (\text{a-vO}_2 \text{ extraction})$$
$$O_2 \text{ pulse} = \dot{V}O_2/\text{HR} = (\text{Stroke volume})$$
$$\times (\text{a-vO}_2 \text{ extraction})$$

Among the three variables contributing to the $\dot{V}O_2$ during a progressive work test, stroke volume remains constant after movement is initiated. For that reason, the normal progressive increase in the O$_2$ pulse during a CPET reflects the progressive increase in a-vO$_2$ extraction as a subject approaches a maximal effort. In the final minute or two of exercise the O$_2$ pulse usually fails to increase, likely secondary to a minimal reduction in stroke volume at the highest possible heart rates (Figure 4.6).

At a maximal cardiovascular effort, the O$_2$ pulse represents a value proportional to the stroke volume, and as with direct measurements of stroke volume, the O$_2$ pulse will be dependent on the size of the subject, with usual values ranging from 8–12 mL/beat for 50-kg subjects to 20–24 mL/beat for 100-kg subjects. An important caution to remember in interpretation of the O$_2$ pulse, however, is that the oxygen content of blood is dependent on hemoglobin concentration, so that the O$_2$ pulse will be reduced in anemic subjects in proportion to the severity of the anemia.

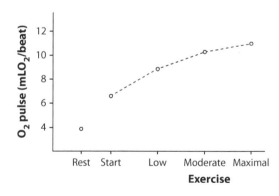

Figure 4.6 Increase in the O$_2$ pulse of a normal subject during a progressive work test.

THE INFLUENCE OF INCREASING BODY TEMPERATURE ON BLOOD-FLOW DISTRIBUTION

Increasing body temperature during exercise will alter the allocation of blood flow, distributing more blood flow to the skin. Muscle is an engine, and similar to any engine, it produces both work and heat. For every 100 watts of power exerted on a cycle ergometer, humans generate over 200 watts of heat. Hence, especially for subjects with a high aerobic capacity, sustained heavy exercise leads to some level of hyperthermia that must be balanced by normal cooling mechanisms. Compared with other animals, we humans have very effective heat-dissipation responses that are achieved by increases in blood flow to the skin and sweating. However the increase in blood flow to the skin for purposes of cooling means that maximal venous extraction of oxygen is reduced, as the blood flow diverted to the skin consumes very little oxygen. The increased allocation of blood flow to the skin during heavy exercise "steals" blood flow from the exercising muscles. Hence, with sustained heavy exercise, particularly in a warm environment, cardiac output will increase to compensate for this diversion of blood flow from exercising muscle. In short-term exercise such as a standard clinical test, this is usually a minor issue, but for subjects capable of very high power outputs during a prolonged test, modest hyperthermia can limit the measured maximal oxygen uptake.

BLOOD PRESSURE RESPONSE DURING A PROGRESSIVE WORK TEST

The normal blood pressure response during a CPET includes a minimal increase in blood pressure in the early stages, followed by a progressive increase in systolic pressures beginning with the onset of exercise-associated metabolic acidosis. Careful monitoring of blood pressure during a progressive work test is an important safety issue. Any failure to increase blood pressure with a heavy exercise load is abnormal and mandates prompt removal of the exercise load, although it is essential to continue leg motion to prevent pooling of blood in the legs. For subjects with poorly controlled hypertension, systolic pressure may exceed 220 mmHg during a test. It is not clear if there is an established upper limit for toleration of exercise hypertension, although systolic pressures of 220 mmHg have been documented in downhill skiers during a race. During post-maximal exercise monitoring, it is important to be aware that unfit young subjects may develop a hypotensive vagal response. If blood pressure shows a rapid drop after a maximal effort, particularly if there is an associated relative bradycardia, those subjects should promptly be moved to a supine posture and kept there for at least 15 minutes before allowing them to sit upright.

PROPERTIES OF HEMOGLOBIN ENHANCING EXERCISE OXYGEN DELIVERY

Hemoglobin is essential for oxygen transport to exercising muscle, but in addition, the properties of the hemoglobin molecule are adapted for exercise to both maximize the oxygen delivery and ameliorate the effects of the CO_2 and hydrogen ion generated within the exercising muscle. The oxygen dissociation curve for hemoglobin has a very steep slope between saturations of 30% and 70%, so that the hemoglobin molecule releases oxygen very readily within exercising muscle in response to small reductions in muscle PO_2 (Figure 4.7).

The oxygen dissociation curve is not fixed but rather can be shifted to the right by three different influences: increases in temperature, hydrogen ion, and CO_2. A right shift of the curve means that, at any given cellular PO_2, more oxygen is released. All three of these influences arise in exercising muscle, although the elevation of muscle temperature is the most important effect causing the right shift of the curve. Hence, arterial blood entering exercising muscle readily releases its oxygen at a relatively higher muscle PO_2 because of these influences. The movement of oxygen from muscle capillary to muscle mitochondria is facilitated by myoglobin within the muscle cells. While myoglobin binds more firmly to oxygen than hemoglobin at any given PO_2, the mitochondrial utilization of oxygen remains fully functional even at partial pressures of oxygen as low as 2–3 mmHg.

Even with the presence of myoglobin within muscle cells, facilitating the transport of oxygen from capillary to mitochondrion, there remains a significant capillary to mitochondrial oxygen partial pressure gradient.

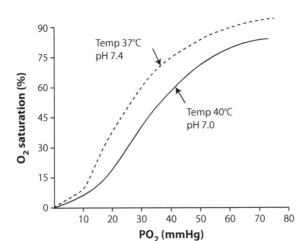

Figure 4.7 Hemoglobin oxygen saturation over the full range of PO_2 values at normal temperature and pH (dotted line) and with the acidosis and hyperthermia typical for blood leaving muscles during heavy exercise (solid line).

This oxygen diffusion limitation within the myocytes represents another limitation to maximal possible oxygen uptake by muscle mitochondria. Well-trained athletes develop both more mitochondria and more extensive capillary networks within their trained muscle groups that reduce the mean diffusion distance. With those long-term muscle training effects, the venous blood exiting the maximally exercising muscles can reach oxygen saturations below 10%.

Hemoglobin also serves an essential role in buffering and removing the CO_2 produced by aerobic metabolism in exercising muscle and the hydrogen ions produced by glycolysis. With the release of oxygen, hemoglobin becomes a better hydrogen ion buffer and, in addition, binds CO_2. Finally within the red blood cell, the enzyme carbonic anhydrase transforms the CO_2 to bicarbonate and hydrogen ion, with the hydrogen ion again more effectively bound by the deoxygenated hemoglobin. Although the PCO_2 in venous blood exiting the exercising muscles may be as high as 70 mmHg, the majority of CO_2 generated by exercising muscle is transported to the heart in the form of bicarbonate.

SUMMARY POINTS

- Maximal exercise capacity in a normal subject during a progressive work test is primarily determined by the maximal cardiac output.
- During a CPET, the heart rate increases linearly with the exercise load and reaches a reproducible maximal exercise heart rate. There is appreciable individual and age-related variability in maximal exercise heart rate.
- The increase in stroke volume during upright exercise is dependent on the effective venous pump that is created when calf muscles contract around the large venous plexuses within the calves. Once leg movement is initiated in a CPET, stroke volume in a normal subject does not increase during the progression to a maximal effort.
- The progressive decrease in mixed venous oxygen during a CPET is a result of progressive direction of blood flow to exercising muscle and reduction of blood flow to renal and splanchnic circulations.
- The progressive increase in O_2 pulse during a progressive work test primarily reflects the nearly linear decrease in mixed venous oxygen saturation throughout the

exercise effort. Maximal O_2 pulse represents both stroke volume and hemoglobin concentration.

- During a CPET, a normal subject will demonstrate a progressive increase in systolic blood pressure most apparent after the onset of the ventilatory threshold.

- Hemoglobin releases oxygen more effectively in the warm and acidotic environment of exercising muscle, and minimizes the acidosis in muscle by binding hydrogen ions. Red blood cell carbonic anhydrase converts the majority of the CO_2 generated within exercising muscle to bicarbonate ion for transport to the lung.

5

Respiratory system during a progressive work test

Ventilation is the first step in the journey of oxygen from the air to its final destination in the mitochondria, and the control of that ventilation during exercise is a complex process controlled by central and peripheral chemosensors and muscle mechanoreceptors. The net effect is that alveolar PO_2 is maintained at a level that ensures full oxygenation of arterial blood. In addition, the maximal capacity of the lung and chest wall system to move air always exceeds the requirements for maximal exercise ventilation, so that, for a normal subject, neither the maximal capacity for exercise ventilation nor exercise gas exchange within the lung will pose limits during a maximal exercise effort. However, the normal respiratory exercise responses described below may be constrained for patients with pulmonary diseases, so it is important to understand the range of normal respiratory responses.

- Alveolar gas measurements during exercise
- Work of breathing during exercise
- Mechanisms controlling exercise ventilation
- Identification of the ventilatory (or anaerobic) threshold
- End-tidal and arterial gas measurements during a CPET
- Pulmonary gas exchange measurements: A-aO_2 difference and V_D/V_T

ALVEOLAR GASES DURING A NORMAL CPET

In the course of a progressive work test, the increases in exercise ventilation must be sufficient to sustain normal levels of alveolar oxygen and carbon dioxide in the face of the progressively increasing cardiac output and the progressive drop in the mixed venous oxygen content in the blood entering the lungs. Commercial exercise testing systems report end-tidal measurements of partial pressures of oxygen and carbon dioxide in the exhaled breath rather than mean alveolar partial pressures, and while those measurements during exercise do not exactly represent the mean alveolar values, they are ordinarily close except during heavy exercise. Those measurements of the alveolar gases during a CPET demonstrate that alveolar ventilation during a maximal effort is more than adequate to maintain normal alveolar partial pressures of oxygen and carbon dioxide, ensuring the normal oxygen content of the arterial blood leaving the lungs (Figure 5.1).

In a normal subject, the end-tidal partial pressures of O_2 and CO_2 provide a good estimate of both alveolar and arterial blood gas partial pressures throughout the exercise effort. Note that, with the onset of heavy exercise, the additional augmentation of ventilation produces an increase in end-tidal PO_2 and a subsequent decrease in end-tidal PCO_2.

WORK OF BREATHING AT REST AND EXERCISE: SPIROMETRY AND MAXIMAL VOLUNTARY VENTILATION (MVV)

Understanding the responses of the lung-chest wall system to the demands of exercise ventilation begins with spirometry before the exercise

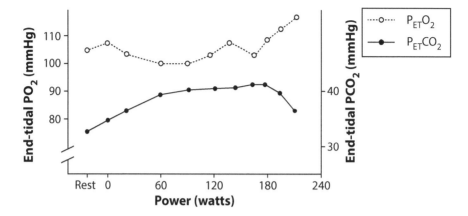

Figure 5.1 Averaged end-tidal measurements of PO_2 and CO_2 in a normal subject during the course of a CPET.

test. Spirometry measurements (illustrated below) start with a normal resting breathing pattern, after which the subject is instructed to inspire to a maximal lung volume, forcibly exhale for at least seven seconds, and then rapidly inspire back to a maximal lung volume (Figure 5.2).

The tidal breaths (before the maximal inhalation) all begin at the lung volume called the functional residual capacity (FRC), which is the volume of gas contained in the lung when all the respiratory muscles are completely relaxed. The inspiratory capacity (IC) is the lung volume that is drawn in with a maximal inspiratory effort beginning from the FRC and ending at the highest possible lung volume, the total lung capacity (TLC). The total volume of gas blown out after the maximal inspiratory effort is the forced vital capacity (FVC), and the fraction of the FVC that is exhaled in the first second is the FEV_1. Following that maximal expiratory effort, there is still gas left in the lung, the residual volume (RV), but that volume cannot be measured with simple spirometry. The final part of the maneuver is a maximal inspiratory effort from RV. Note that the final part of the FVC

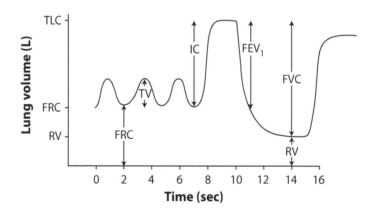

Figure 5.2 Conduct of a spirometry measurement, beginning with tidal breathing, followed by a maximal inspiratory effort, a maximal expiratory effort, and a maximal inspiratory effort from residual volume. TV is the tidal volume of normal breathing, and functional residual capacity (FRC) is the lung volume at the beginning of a normal breath. Inspiratory capacity (IC) is the volume inspired from FRC with a maximal inspiratory effort, reaching the total lung capacity (TLC). The vital capacity (VC) is the maximal volume of gas that can be exhaled from TLC, and FEV_1 is the volume expired in the first second of the VC effort. The residual volume (RV) is the gas remaining in the lung after a maximal expiratory effort.

effort brings lung volume below the FRC to the RV, and reaching that lower lung volume requires expiratory muscular effort. A normal FEV_1 will be 70%–80% of the FVC, depending on the age of the subject.

Measurements from spirometry of maximal expiration and inspiration are usually presented graphically as a flow-volume loop, and this presentation is helpful to picture the respiratory pattern changes during exercise. Both the forced vital capacity maneuver and the forced inspiratory effort are measurements of volume changes over time. Volume per unit of time is a flow, and the expiratory and inspiratory flow efforts can be plotted against lung volume from the total lung capacity (TLC) to the residual volume (RV), with the upper expiratory loop moving from TLC to RV and the lower inspiratory loop from RV back to TLC (Figure 5.3).

The maximal expiratory loop shows the highest flow at the very beginning of the expiratory effort (at total lung capacity), with the majority of that volume exhaled within the first second. The progressively decreasing flows in the final several seconds of forced exhalation reflect the progressive increases in small airways resistance with reductions in lung volume. Because of the increasing airways resistance as lung volume decreases, the expiratory flows in the final two-thirds of the expiratory loop are independent of muscular effort. The maximal inspiratory loop on the bottom is a different shape, as those inspiratory flows are determined primarily by muscular effort. The smaller tidal volume loop, representing normal resting ventilation, starts at the FRC and has much lower inspiratory and expiratory flow rates.

The final pulmonary function measurement needed before an exercise test is the maximal voluntary ventilation (MVV). The subject is coached to take the deepest, fastest breaths possible for 12 seconds, and the total amount of gas exhaled in that 12-second period is multiplied by five, giving an MVV measurement in units of liters per minute (Figure 5.4).

During a well-performed MVV maneuver, the maximal inspiratory volume is just below the IC, and the exhalation volume is below the FRC. For normal subjects, an acceptable MVV effort (in liters per minute) is about 40 times the measured FEV_1. The MVV measurement represents a resting measurement of the maximal ventilatory capacity, which is used for later comparison with

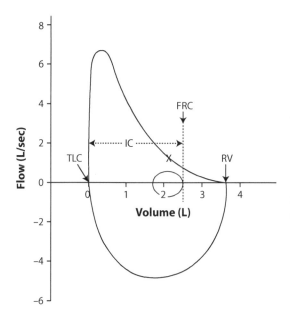

Figure 5.3 A flow-volume loop with flow on the ordinate and volume on the abscissa. Maximal expiratory flow (upper line) and maximal inspiratory flow (lower line) measurements produce the flow-volume loop. The "X" on the expiratory loop marks the volume exhaled in the first second (FEV_1). The small loop inside the maximal flow volume loop represents the inspiratory and expiratory flows seen during normal tidal breathing. The vertical dashed line at the exhalation end of the tidal volume loop marks the functional residual capacity (FRC), and the horizontal dashed line represents the inspiratory capacity (IC).

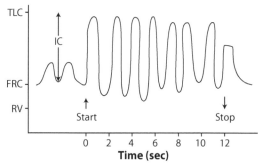

Figure 5.4 Maximal voluntary ventilation, measured during a 12-second maximal breathing effort. MVV is the total exhaled volume from the 12-second effort, FRC is the resting volume for normal breathing, and IC is the inspiratory capacity measured during prior spirometry.

the ventilation achieved during a maximal exercise effort.

WORK OF BREATHING AT REST AND EXERCISE: EXERCISE VENTILATION DURING A CPET

At maximal effort, the volume of gas inhaled per minute (termed minute ventilation) that is required to maintain a normal alveolar PO_2 never reaches the MVV that was measured at rest. For most normal subjects giving a maximal effort, maximal exercise ventilation requires no more than 65%–75% of the MVV. Thus, any normal subject reaching a maximal exercise effort, if instructed to breathe more, can do so. In short, normal subjects do not experience a ventilatory limitation when giving a maximal effort during a progressive work test (Figure 5.5).

The increase in ventilation during a progressive work test requires increases in both tidal volume and respiratory rate. In the early stages of exercise, the increase in ventilation comes mostly from increases in tidal volume, but once the exercise tidal volume approaches 60%–70% of the vital capacity, the additional increases in minute ventilation come primarily from increases in respiratory rate. The relative limitation of vital capacity breathing during heavy exercise represents a strategy to limit the work of breathing, as explained below in the description of lung compliance (Figure 5.6).

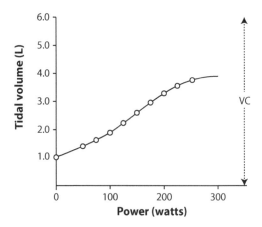

Figure 5.6 Increases in tidal volume during the conduct of a CPET, plotted against power output. The vertical line represents the volume of a vital capacity breath.

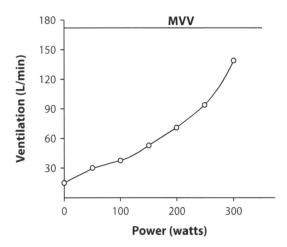

Figure 5.5 Maximal exercise ventilation is less than the MVV.

Work of breathing at rest and exercise: Lung compliance

The elastic properties of the lungs and the chest wall balance at FRC, with the balance reflecting the chest wall attempting to spring open and the lungs attempting to collapse. The lung volume at FRC constitutes the lung volume in which the least effort is required to inspire a breath of a given volume. A pressure-volume curve of the lung and chest wall system represents the properties of that system when no muscular effort is expended (Figure 5.7).

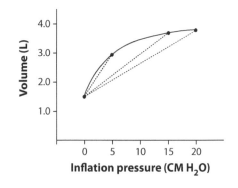

Figure 5.7 Inflation pressures required to inflate a relaxed intact lung and chest wall to three different tidal volumes.

From this diagram, it is apparent that fully inflating the lung requires far more inflation pressure (or inspiratory muscle work) than the pressures needed to do smaller inflations. Inspired volumes greater than about 60% of the inspiratory capacity add disproportionately to the work of breathing. As noted above, nearly all subjects with normal lungs will limit their tidal volumes to around 60% of their forced vital capacity during heavy exercise. The muscular work of ventilation required during moderate exercise has been estimated to require about 3% of the exercise oxygen consumption. At the highest levels of exercise ventilation, airways resistance to the high inspiratory and expiratory flows add to the respiratory muscular work, possibly accounting for as much as 8%–10% of the maximal oxygen consumption.

Work of breathing at rest and exercise: Using the flow-volume loop

The flow-volume loop measured at rest before an exercise test provides a baseline for superimposed exercise flow-volume loops to illustrate how the areas of lung capacity are used during a maximal exercise effort (Figure 5.8). Flow-volume loops during exercise provide useful insights into limitations for patients with airflow obstruction.

Despite the increased volume and rate of breathing with maximal effort, expiratory flow rates do not exceed the resting maximal expiratory flow-volume loop. For subjects with normal pulmonary function, the final fraction of exhaled tidal volume during exercise finishes below the resting FRC, and the maximal tidal inspiration during exercise does not reach the total lung capacity. Thus, a full inspiratory capacity effort during exercise is larger than the resting IC measurement because each exercise breath begins below the resting FRC. The inspiratory capacity can be measured during exercise by the same procedure described for

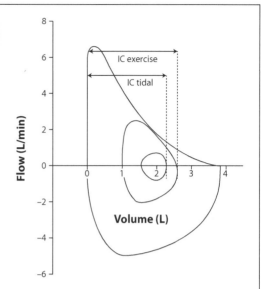

Figure 5.8 Flow-volume loop at rest (smallest loop) and heavy exercise flow-volume loop (middle loop), within the maximal expiratory and inspiratory loop measured before exercise. IC tidal and IC exercise represent the different inspiratory capacities measured at rest and exercise.

spirometry. The patient is instructed to make a maximal inspiratory effort after a normal exercise exhalation. Inspiratory capacity can be measured periodically throughout an exercise test and normally will show a modest increase during exercise, reflecting the lower lung volume reached at the beginning of a breath during heavy exercise. The exercise inspiratory capacity will always be bigger than the maximal exercise tidal volume because of the extra inspiratory effort needed to reach total lung capacity.

NEURAL DETERMINANTS OF EXERCISE VENTILATION

The stability of arterial oxygen saturation measurements over the normal eight- to fifteen-fold increase in oxygen consumption during an exercise test requires a strong correlation between the entry of fresh gas into the lung and the oxygen requirements of the exercising muscle. Several factors contribute to the appropriate ventilatory response to progressive exercise. Immediately on initiation of exercise, cortical input initiates the ventilation response, and this is further augmented by afferent neural signals from the exercising muscles and joints. As exercise progresses, neural output from both the brainstem and carotid sinus adjust the exercise ventilation volume to maintain a constant arterial PCO_2. With the onset of heavy exercise and associated acidosis and elevated norepinephrine from exercising muscle, those two sensory systems provide additional stimulation to ventilation, causing the arterial PCO_2 to drop below the resting value to partially compensate for the exercise acidosis. In the abnormal setting of arterial hypoxemia developing during exercise, that change is sensed in the carotid sinus, which then provides an additional stimulus to further increase exercise ventilation.

Given the multiple neural systems contributing to exercise ventilation, it is not surprising that there are substantial differences among normal subjects in the amount of minute ventilation used for a given level of work. Two CPET measurements that represent those inter-individual differences in exercise ventilation sensitivity are the ratio between exercise ventilation and oxygen consumption (the ventilatory equivalent for oxygen, $\dot{V}E/\dot{V}O_2$) and the ratio between ventilation and CO_2 production (the ventilatory equivalent for CO_2, $\dot{V}E/\dot{V}CO_2$) (Figure 5.9).

For estimation of exercise ventilation sensitivity, the values of either ratio are averaged before the ventilatory threshold is reached. Individuals with blunted ventilatory sensitivity will have $\dot{V}E/\dot{V}O_2$ ratios of around 20 liters/liter, and individuals with high sensitivity will have $\dot{V}E/\dot{V}O_2$ ratios of around 33 liters/liter. These different exercise ventilation sensitivities appear to be inherited and are not appreciably altered by either training or

sedentary lifestyle. Normal subjects with high ventilatory sensitivity still do not have a ventilatory limitation to maximal exercise, although they may be more likely to describe shortness of breath during a maximal effort.

IDENTIFICATION OF THE VENTILATORY (OR ANAEROBIC) THRESHOLD

Clinical interpretation of a progressive work test requires the identification of the time during a test when the metabolic acidosis of exercise becomes manifest, the point described as the ventilatory (or anaerobic) threshold. This point can be identified by examination of the CPET measurements of ventilation and gas exchange. The increase in arterial lactate concentrations during the final stages of a CPET reflects the onset of muscle norepinephrine release and glycolysis in the heavily exercising muscles, with the associated metabolic acidosis and supplemental ATP production. As noted in the muscle chapter, the beginning of this metabolic acidosis could be best identified during a CPET with multiple arterial blood samples drawn for lactate concentrations. However a ventilatory threshold can ordinarily be identified noninvasively by the onset of an additional increase in exercise ventilation, hence the term ventilatory threshold. There are three CPET measurements that assist in the identification of the exercise ventilatory threshold, and ordinarily all three should be considered for a best consensus estimate (Figure 5.10).

The V-slope estimate plots CO_2 output on the Y-axis versus O_2 consumption on the X-axis. In most tests, it appears that the plot resembles two lines with different slopes that intersect at 40%–55% of the maximal O_2 consumption. That oxygen consumption at the intersection of the two lines is one representation of the ventilatory (or anaerobic) threshold. The V-slope estimate ordinarily best reflects the onset of the arterial blood lactate increase during a CPET, but the estimate can be difficult to identify in patients with irregular exercise breathing patterns. An advantage of the V-slope estimate is that it can be objectively identified by the software in most exercise systems, although the graphical plot should be examined to confirm that fit. The location of a V-slope ventilatory threshold in an exercise study always arises about 10% earlier in the exercise effort compared with the locations

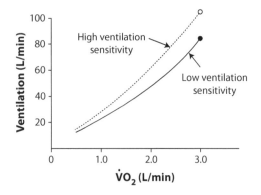

Figure 5.9 Plots of $\dot{V}E$ vs. $\dot{V}O_2$ for two subjects with different exercise ventilation sensitivity.

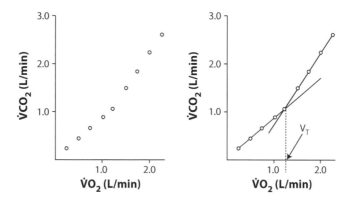

Figure 5.10 The V-slope estimate plots paired measurements of $\dot{V}O_2$ (X-axis) and $\dot{V}CO_2$ (Y-axis) collected during the CPET (left graph). Two straight lines are drawn (right graph), one adjusted to the initial portion of exercise effort and the other set to the final effort. The intersection of the two lines (marked with the vertical line) represents the ventilatory threshold (V_T) identified by the V-slope method.

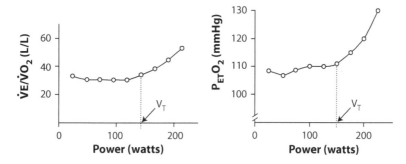

Figure 5.11 Plots of ventilatory equivalent for O_2 ($\dot{V}E/\dot{V}O_2$) against power output (left graph) and end-tidal PO_2 against power output (right graph). Ventilatory thresholds are identified with vertical dotted lines.

identified from increases in end-tidal PO_2 ($P_{ET}O_2$) and $\dot{V}E/\dot{V}O_2$ (Figure 5.11).

The next estimate of the ventilatory threshold is based on the progression of exercise changes in the ventilatory equivalent for O_2 ($\dot{V}E/\dot{V}O_2$). $\dot{V}E/\dot{V}O_2$ values (left graph) are relatively constant in early exercise and are followed until a clear increase is noted, representing the ventilatory threshold. The estimate from the graph should be confirmed with trends seen in the tabular 20-second data printout, choosing the best estimate of when the value begins to increase and fails to return to the original baseline. The other estimate of the ventilatory threshold uses the end-tidal O_2 measurement (right graph), a value that again becomes relatively constant in early exercise until the onset of the acidosis of heavy exercise. With this acidosis, there is compensatory hyperventilation producing a progressive increase in end-tidal O_2, marking this estimate of a ventilatory threshold. With both the $\dot{V}E/\dot{V}O_2$ and end-tidal PO_2 estimates, subjects may show some oscillation of the respective values at the onset of the ventilatory threshold, so an optimal identification of the ventilatory threshold by these two markers may have a subjective component.

The $P_{ET}O_2$, and $\dot{V}E/\dot{V}O_2$ estimates tend to agree and both come somewhat later in the exercise effort than the V-slope estimate, at 60%–70% of the exercise effort. A ventilatory equivalent estimate using CO_2 ($\dot{V}E/\dot{V}CO_2$) begins to increase *after* the three estimates described above and is not used as a marker of the ventilatory threshold. Likewise, the time during the exercise test when the respiratory R value exceeds 1.0 should not be used as a determinant of the ventilatory threshold, as that point may be reached on, before, or after the three accepted markers.

End-tidal gas measurements during a progressive work test

The measurements of PO_2 and PCO_2 reported by standard exercise systems are end-tidal measurements, not average alveolar values. End-tidal sampling was developed over a century ago to obtain a sample representing the average gas composition of the alveolar spaces, avoiding the initial part of an exhalation from the upper airways, where no gas exchange takes place. Breath-by-breath measurements made by current exercise systems accurately measure gas concentrations throughout the entire exhaled breath, and all of those measurements are used for calculation of oxygen consumption and carbon dioxide output for each breath. However the gas concentrations reported by all commercial breath-by-breath exercise systems represent only a sample of the final portion of each exhaled breath and do not reflect the true mean alveolar gas concentrations during heavy exercise (Figure 5.12).

Figure 5.12 illustrates changes during a single exhalation in PO_2 and PCO_2, measured at the mouth. Note that, at rest, once the inspired gas that resided in the upper airways has been exhaled, the gas concentrations are nearly constant. For a normal subject at rest (left plot above), the end-tidal PCO_2 is usually a reasonable estimate of the arterial PCO_2. The end-tidal PO_2 at rest may be slightly higher than the arterial PO_2 for reasons discussed below. During heavy exercise, however, because of the eight- to fifteen-fold increase in O_2 and CO_2 exchange and the three- to four-fold increase in tidal volume, there are then wide swings in gas concentration in the alveolar spaces in the course of a single exhalation (Figure 5.12, right plot). While the exercise measurements of *arterial* PO_2 and PCO_2 reflect an average of these fluctuating alveolar gas values during heavy exercise, the end-tidal CO_2 will exceed both the average alveolar PCO_2 and the arterial PCO_2, and the opposite effect will be present with the end-tidal PO_2, which will be lower than the mean alveolar PO_2. The end-tidal measurements of PO_2 are very helpful for identification of a ventilatory threshold, but do not accurately reflect either mean alveolar or arterial PO_2 during heavy exercise. The end-tidal measurements of CO_2 during heavy exercise overestimate the average arterial PCO_2 by as much as 6 mmHg.

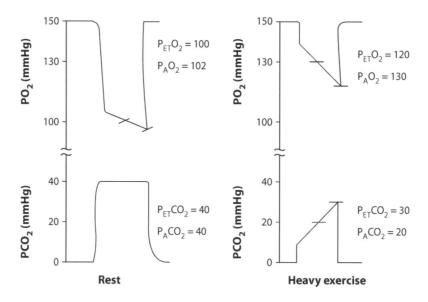

Figure 5.12 Normal within-breath swings of end-tidal PO_2 and PCO_2 measured at the mouth at rest (left plot) and during heavy exercise (right plot).

PULMONARY GAS EXCHANGE DURING A PROGRESSIVE WORK TEST

The efficiency of exchange of O_2 and CO_2 in a normal lung during exercise is described by the very small differences noted between the mean alveolar partial pressures of the two gases and the arterial partial pressures. The figure below shows arterial and alveolar partial pressures for both O_2 and CO_2 in a normal subject undergoing a progressive work test (Figure 5.13).

The mean alveolar PO_2 is calculated from the CPET measurements of CO_2 output and O_2 consumption and the arterial $PaCO_2$ (see description below). Unlike the mean alveolar PO_2, which increases progressively after the ventilatory threshold, the arterial PO_2 remains unchanged throughout a progressive work test. The normal value for the alveolar PO_2 to arterial PO_2 difference (A-a DO_2) at rest is 7–15 mmHg and with exercise remains unchanged until the subject approaches maximal effort, at which time a modest increase in A-a DO_2 develops, but it still is ordinarily less than 20 mmHg. Because of the within-breath changes in gas concentrations during exercise described earlier, the maximal exercise end-tidal PO_2 measurement is lower than the true mean alveolar PO_2 and cannot be used for the calculation of the alveolar PO_2 to arterial PO_2 difference.

Research studies with more sophisticated gas exchange measurements have shown that the

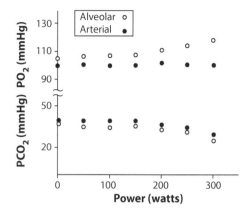

Figure 5.13 The time course of changes in alveolar and arterial values of PO_2 and PCO_2 in a normal subject during a CPET. During heavy exercise, the difference between alveolar and arterial PO_2 increases, while the alveolar and arterial values for CO_2 remain close.

increased A-a O_2 difference at maximal exercise is attributable to an increase in the normal degree of mismatch between blood flow and ventilation in the lung, an increase in the overall extent of ventilation-perfusion heterogeneity. A second cause of an increased A-a O_2 difference seen in some subjects with exceptionally high exercise cardiac outputs is an oxygen diffusion limitation. For those individuals, at maximal exercise, the residence time for blood in the lung is so short that there is not adequate time for the erythrocytes to become fully oxygenated.

Gas exchange calculations: Arterial-alveolar difference

The arterial-alveolar difference is a calculation that represents the effects of mismatch between ventilation and blood flow within the lung, and it is abnormal in nearly all parenchymal lung diseases and also cardiac disorders that include right-to-left shunts. The calculation requires an arterial blood gas sample for measurements of PO_2 and PCO_2 and exercise system measurements of CO_2 output ($\dot{V}CO_2$) and O_2 consumption ($\dot{V}O_2$). The latter two measurements are used to calculate the respiratory R value ($R = \dot{V}CO_2/\dot{V}O_2$). The inspired PO_2 (PIO_2) of

completely humidified inspired gas at a barometric pressure of 760 mmHg is 149 mmHg. $PIO_2 = 0.21*(760 - 47)$. (The 47 mmHg term represents the tracheal water vapor pressure of water at 37° centigrade.) The average alveolar PO_2 (PAO_2) is then calculated as follows:

$$PAO_2 = PIO_2 - PaCO_2/R$$

Finally, the arterial PO_2 (PaO_2) is used to calculate the A-a difference

$$\text{A-a } O_2 \text{ difference} = PAO_2 - PaO_2$$

Gas exchange calculations: Physiologic dead space

A second measurement of gas exchange efficiency during a progressive work test is the physiologic dead space. In normal subjects, most dead space ventilation represents the portion of an inspired breath that never goes deeper than the conducting airways. The volume of this anatomic dead space in cubic centimeters is roughly equivalent to a subject's ideal body weight in pounds. At rest, that fraction of anatomic dead space in an exhaled breath is around 30% of the exhalation. However, with exercise, as the tidal volume increases progressively, the anatomic dead space represents a progressively smaller fraction of each exhaled breath. However, the physiologic dead space includes not only this anatomic dead space component, but also the contribution to wasted ventilation from mismatch between alveolar ventilation and blood flow. In normal subjects, this contribution is quite small, but in nearly all pulmonary and pulmonary vascular diseases, the mismatch within the lung between ventilation and capillary blood flow is substantially larger and therefore increases the calculated physiologic dead space (Figure 5.14).

Calculation of physiologic dead space

A modification of the original Bohr dead space equation is used to calculate the physiologic dead space. This physiologic dead space measurement includes both the anatomic dead space influence described above plus the influence of mismatch between ventilation and blood flow in the lung. In normal subjects during exercise, this mismatch influence is a small contribution compared to the anatomic dead space effect. However, with nearly all lung diseases, regions of diseased lung with high VA/Q ratios make a major contribution to the wasted ventilation calculation and provide important information for interpretation of an exercise study. The physiologic dead space equation requires an arterial PCO_2 measurement and a mixed expired CO_2 measurement

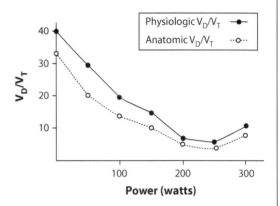

Figure 5.14 Changes in anatomic dead space (open dots) shown as a fraction of tidal volume during a CPET, compared with measurements of physiologic dead space (closed dots).

(P_ECO_2) obtained from the exercise measurements of minute ventilation ($\dot{V}E$, L/min) and CO_2 ($\dot{V}CO_2$, L/min) output obtained at the time the blood gas was drawn.

$$P_ECO_2(mmHg) = (\dot{V}CO_2/\dot{V}E) \times 863(mmHg)$$

(The constant 863 mmHg is needed instead of the standard sea-level 760 mmHg for atmospheric pressure because the $\dot{V}CO_2$ is described at standard temperature [273 K] and the $\dot{V}E$ is described at body temperature [310 K].)

$$V_D/V_T = (PaCO_2 - P_ECO_2)/PaCO_2$$

The normal progression of the physiologic dead space measurement during exercise is illustrated above in Figure 5.13. Note that it parallels the anatomic dead space changes for this normal subject. While a normal maximal exercise value for physiologic V_D/V_T is quoted as less than 20%, most normal subjects during exercise will have values less than 10%.

Commercial exercise systems present a calculation of V_D/V_T, but that calculation uses the end-tidal PCO_2 measurement in place of arterial PCO_2, and as described above concerning end-tidal measurement, during exercise, this yields an inappropriately high estimate of the physiologic dead space, as the exercise end-tidal PCO_2 can exceed the arterial PCO_2 by 6 mmHg or more in a normal subject. The net result of using the end-tidal PCO_2 measurement instead of the (correct) arterial PCO_2 measurement in the physiologic dead space calculation for a normal subject is that the calculated physiologic dead space will be too high. For subjects with pulmonary diseases, the opposite problem arises, as end-tidal PCO_2 is often substantially below arterial PCO_2 and the calculated physiologic dead space will be too low.

SUMMARY POINTS

- Throughout a progressive exercise test, normal subjects maintain a normal PaO_2, although a small increase in the A-a O_2 difference develops with maximal effort.
- The exercise performance of a normal subject undergoing a CPET is not limited by ventilatory capacity. Maximal exercise ventilation in normal subjects is 20%–30% less than their maximal voluntary ventilation measured at rest.
- During a progressive exercise test, normal subjects increase ventilation by increases in both tidal volume and respiratory rate until they reach an exercise tidal volume of roughly 60% of their vital capacity. After that point, additional increases in exercise ventilation are achieved by rate increases alone.
- The ventilatory threshold identifies the onset of exercise metabolic acidosis and is identified by the V-slope graph or by increases in the end-tidal PO_2 or the increases in the ventilatory equivalent for oxygen ($\dot{V}E/\dot{V}O_2$).
- After the onset of the metabolic acidosis of heavy exercise, normal subjects develop progressive compensatory hyperventilation, leading to decreases in both arterial and end-tidal PCO_2.
- Arterial blood gases, although not ordinarily obtained during a routine CPET, are helpful in a number of diagnostic investigations in which exercise measurements of A-aO_2 difference and physiologic dead space will add useful information for interpretation of the test results.

6

Planning and conducting the exercise test

A cardiopulmonary exercise test can be performed competently under the supervision of a well-trained technician, but those test findings are far more useful if they can be interpreted within the context of a patient's medical history. Hence, the information gathered before the performance of the test is an irreplaceable part of optimal test interpretation. This chapter discusses the information that will assist in that interpretation.

- Determine why the test was requested
- Obtain an exercise-relevant medical history
- Assess exercise risks
- Select an exercise mode and exercise increments
- Patient orientation to a CPET
- Measurements before the CPET
- System setup and preparation for the patient
- Monitoring measurements during the test
- Patient safety during the test
- Exercise recovery

DETERMINE WHY THE TEST WAS REQUESTED

The average health care provider does not ordinarily order a CPET as a diagnostic test, so when a request for a CPET is received, it usually means that something unexpected has developed with a patient's exercise-related symptoms. The reasons for CPET requests usually fall within three general categories.

The first is where the cause of the exercise limitation is uncertain, and the aim of the study is to gain both an objective assessment of the overall limitation and to identify an organ-specific exercise pattern of that limited response. This category includes studies on competitive athletes who have lost exercise tolerance and may arrive at a diagnosis of overtraining syndrome, in which case followup CPETs will be help to guide recovery. Additionally, CPET is often helpful to characterize an aerobic athletes potential or progress of training.

The second category of test request is for patients with a known exercise-limiting diagnosis, but where the overall impairment is more severe than appears attributable to that disorder or when the expected response to treatment has failed to develop.

The final category of CPET request is to follow the maximal oxygen uptake of patients with severe heart failure or adult congenital heart disease to identify the appropriate timing for consideration of advanced heart failure treatments such as transplantation or installation of a cardiac assist device. Even within that final category, however, relevant new diagnostic information may be gained from the CPET interpretation.

OBTAIN AN EXERCISE-RELEVANT MEDICAL HISTORY

Because of the wide range of exercise tolerance among normal subjects, it is important to learn about the patient's exercise capacity before the development of symptoms. An exercise baseline is relatively easy to estimate for persons whose occupations require sustained heavy physical activity or for persons who participate in competitive sports or any recreational activities sufficient to cause sweating. For the resolutely sedentary person, however, some sense of baseline aerobic capacity can be obtained from their prior ability to perform sustained everyday exercise tasks such as vacuuming large rooms, mowing a lawn, or ability to do sustained uphill walks. Questions about activities that require several minutes of exercise are better for estimation of exercise capacity than examples of very short-term exercise such as stair climbing. For patients undergoing a follow-up CPET, their perception of change in exercise tolerance since the last test is also helpful. The onset and progression of the exercise-limiting symptoms over time may be diagnostically helpful. As examples, a waxing and waning symptom of dyspnea over time is more suggestive of asthma or hypersensitivity pneumonitis, a progressive stepwise increase in dyspnea might raise concern for pulmonary embolism, and a slow loss of exercise capacity with generalized fatigue and cold intolerance might suggest hypothyroidism.

Patients sent for a diagnostic CPET ordinarily have had prior diagnostic studies performed, usually including basic laboratory measurements, pulmonary function tests, and echocardiography. Those findings should be reviewed. For all patients, it is helpful to have measurements of hemoglobin concentration and thyroid stimulating hormone.

ASSESS EXERCISE RISK

A progressive work exercise protocol continued to a maximal effort involves unacceptable risks in a few clinical situations. The most obvious contraindication is a recent myocardial infarction or a symptomatic history suggestive of unstable angina. Once a myocardial infarction has healed and the patient stabilized on appropriate treatment including beta blockade, then a CPET may be performed with acceptable safety. Likewise for patients with severe heart failure, after pharmacologic treatment has been optimized and, if indicated, an implanted defibrillator is placed, a CPET may be performed with acceptable risk. However patients who have experienced exercise-induced syncope represent an exceptionally high-risk group that should not be subjected to a maximal effort CPET. This latter group includes patients with severe pulmonary hypertension, tight aortic stenosis, and obstructive myocardial hypertrophy.

CHOOSING AN EXERCISE MODE AND EXERCISE INCREMENTS

Although either cycle ergometer or treadmill exercise are appropriate for CPET assessment, there are differences that may guide the choice.

For the majority of patients tested, a maximal effort on a treadmill will yield an oxygen uptake that is about 10% higher than a maximal effort on a cycle ergometer, and the treadmill test will also produce a slightly higher maximal heart rate. For patients with chronotropic impairment and implanted motion-detecting pacemakers, the arm swing and/or impact of treadmill exercise is required to trigger a faster heart rate. However, a treadmill CPET that must include mask apparatus, blood pressure cuff, oximeter, and electrode attachments is more challenging for subjects, particularly if they are apprehensive, frail, or confused. The latter patients in particular are more safely monitored on a cycle ergometer. In addition, the cycle ergometer provides a reliable measurement of power output to match against the measured oxygen consumption.

The treadmill protocol chosen for a given patient should provide at least 10 minutes of exercise data. For patients with severe exercise impairment, the original Bruce treadmill protocol may not be tolerated for more that four or five minutes, and a short exercise duration can make test interpretation more challenging. A better choice for more exercise-impaired patients is the modified Naughton protocol that uses a more limited treadmill speed, not exceeding a 3.5-mph walk, with increases in exercise load achieved by progressive treadmill elevation. An experienced clinician can also customize each test on the treadmill, aiming to achieve about 10 minutes of data prior to exhaustion. For a customized protocol, recognize that an adult can walk briskly at 3.5–4 mph before having to jog, and if faster speeds are planned, it is important to confirm that the patient is able to jog or run. The treadmill protocol used must be specifically described in the exercise report to permit a comparable exercise stress for follow-up exercise studies.

To achieve a 10-minute exercise effort on an ergometer, the size of the subject must be taken into account when choosing the rate for the watt increments. The important difference between ergometer and treadmill protocols is that, on a treadmill, the subject is carrying his or her own weight, so that a 6-foot, 4-inch male and a 5-foot woman could be exercised using the same treadmill speed and grade protocol. However, on an ergometer, those two normal subjects might require 25-watt and 10-watt ergometer increments per minute, respectively, to complete a test lasting 10 minutes, as a larger subject is able to achieve a larger absolute power output. Additional downward adjustments in watt increment need to be made for the most disabled patients, and accomplished aerobic athletes may require higher increments, but the subject size is always an important consideration in the choice of ergometer power increments. The electronically braked ergometers can provide constant work increments that are relatively independent of pedal speed, although we ordinarily instruct the patients to maintain a pedal speed in the 60–70 rpm range throughout the test.

PATIENT ORIENTATION TO A CPET

To assure full patient involvement, we review the exercise-relevant medical history with the patient before the test and ask about their concerns relative to the testing. A maximal exercise test is a team effort involving the patient, the physician, and the respiratory technician. It is the only medical test that requires a symptom-limited maximal effort from the patient, and for that reason, it is essential for the patient to understand both the medical rationale for giving that effort and the safety precautions that will be employed. We explain to the patient that they should discontinue the exercise effort if they develop lightheadedness or severe chest pain, but that otherwise they will be encouraged to give a maximal effort at the end of the test. We also explain that we will stop the test if we observe serious cardiac arrhythmias or find that their blood pressure is failing to increase in a normal fashion with heavy exercise. Finally, we review the risks of maximal exercise testing, including the very distant probabilities of serious cardiac arrhythmia and death, and obtain written consent to perform the test.

For patients exercised on a cycle ergometer, we explain that a maximal effort has been attained when they are no longer able to consistently sustain a pedal rate greater than 60 rpm. For patients exercised on a treadmill, a maximal effort is attained when they have to grab the handrails with both hands to keep up with the treadmill speed and grade. If measurements of subjective exertion during the test are desired, we explain to the patient how to rate their fatigue on a Borg scale by pointing to number on the scale.

MEASUREMENTS BEFORE THE CPET

On the day of the test, a resting ECG is recorded and reviewed to rule out any suggestion of acute ischemic changes and to compare the ECG with previously obtained tracings. Spirometry measurements are repeated on the day of the test, including a maximal flow-volume loop that can be used with some exercise systems to superimpose on exercise flow-volume loops. Finally, a 12-second measurement of maximal voluntary ventilation is acquired to assist with interpretation of the maximal exercise ventilation response.

Exercise arterial blood gases are an important addition to a diagnostic CPET if the clinical history suggests either possible exercise-associated desaturation or that pulmonary vascular disease or interstitial lung disease are among the potential diagnostic considerations. While some clinicians prefer to insert a radial artery catheter for secure blood sampling throughout the test, others have been satisfied with an immediate post-exercise arterial sample by radial artery puncture. With either choice, the necessary equipment for arterial sampling needs to be assembled before the exercise portion of the test, and that part of the test needs to be explained to the patient.

SYSTEM SETUP AND PREPARATION FOR THE PATIENT

Prior to the test, the technician calibrates both the gas analysis and respiratory flow devices of the CPET system and sets the exercise system software for the desired exercise increments. It is essential to recognize that a capable and motivated laboratory technician is the most important determinant of a successful CPET. Beyond the competence to operate the exercise testing apparatus, the best technicians have the enthusiasm and interpersonal skills to help their patients give their best efforts during the testing. The technician explains the ergometer or treadmill protocol to the patient while placing the standard 12 ECG leads on the patient. The ergometer seat height is adjusted for the patient and the exercise goal of maintaining a pedal speed between 60 and 70 rpm for as long as possible is explained. The patient is told the test will be stopped when they are no longer able to maintain a pedal speed above 60 rpm. If a treadmill protocol is planned, the patient is told that they may keep one hand on the bar at the front of the treadmill during exercise, but when they have to grab the bar with both hands, the test is over, and the treadmill will immediately be slowed to a stop. After the exercise device orientation, with the patient seated on the ergometer or standing on the treadmill, the blood pressure cuff, oximeter probe, and face mask (or mouth piece and nose clips) are adjusted to the patient.

MONITORING MEASUREMENTS DURING THE TEST

The initial data collection during the patient rest period while on the cycle ergometer or the treadmill is primarily an opportunity to check all of the components of the exercise system, including the ECG screen, the oximeter pulse tracing and gas exchange measurements. The respiratory exchange ratio (R, $\dot{V}CO_2/\dot{V}O_2$) should stabilize in a reasonable range (roughly between 0.75 and 0.85). Values below that range may suggest that gas calibration should be rechecked, and values above that range are usually associated with subject hyperventilation but could also suggest gas calibration problems. If significant hyperventilation persists during this three-minute period to collect resting measurements, it is helpful for subsequent test interpretation to prolong the time for unloaded pedaling (or slow, level walking on the treadmill) until the R value drops back into the expected range before initiating the progressive work protocol.

Assuming that any initial hyperventilation has resolved, following the increase of respiratory R values during the progressive work portion of the test provides an opportunity to anticipate when the patient will reach a maximal cardiovascular effort. The point during the test when respiratory R exceeds 1.0 is near the ventilatory threshold and suggests that the subject is somewhere between two-thirds to three-quarters through their maximal effort. This point is also associated with an appreciable increase in systolic blood pressure. When the R exceeds 1.0, it is helpful to tell the subject that you know they are working hard and to begin coaching them to continue their effort as long as possible.

PATIENT SAFETY DURING THE TEST

Continued direct observation of the patient during exercise is crucial in ensuring patient safety. While the physician should coach the subject to give their best effort and not to be deterred by leg fatigue or shortness of breath, symptoms such as chest pain, lightheadedness, or confusion during heavy exercise are valid criteria for stopping the test. Blood pressure should be measured at least every two minutes throughout the test. While the systolic pressure may drop modestly between rest and the initial exercise stages, a progressive increase in systolic pressures is expected during the final exercise stages, and any decrease in systolic pressure during heavy effort mandates stopping the test. In that setting, the patient should be instructed to maintain unloaded pedaling (or stepping in place once the treadmill has stopped), and blood pressure should be monitored each minute until it normalizes. High systolic pressures with maximal effort are not an indication for stopping a test.

Both the physician and technician should monitor the ECG tracings during and after the exercise effort. Ventricular premature contractions (VPCs) noted during rest or early exercise that vanish as work load progresses are almost always benign, but VPCs that develop during heavy exercise are not. The decision to stop a test based on exercise-associated VPCs is easier to make with the understanding that patients demonstrating multifocal VPCs or bigeminy during heavy exercise are likely to show even more ectopy after exercise is stopped. During exercise, the development of 2-mm of downsloping ST depression in the anterior leads or the development of exercise-associated bundle branch block are highly suggestive of significant coronary artery disease, and ordinarily the exercise phase of the test should be stopped at that point. Finally, the onset of any broad complex tachycardia during exercise should be assumed to be ventricular tachycardia and the test stopped. Although subsequent study of those exercise ECG tracings and the following exercise recovery tracings usually reveals bundle branch block or supraventricular tachycardia with aberrant conduction, those calls cannot be made with any confidence in the midst of an exercise test.

Oximeter readings during exercise can be misleading, particularly if the oximeter monitor does not show a consistent pulse waveform. Patients with true pulmonary gas exchange abnormalities or an intracardiac shunt will show a gradual progression of desaturation as the workload increases, and with the cessation of exercise, the oxygen saturation will remain abnormal in the first minute of recovery. If the arterial oxygen saturation (SaO_2) drops abruptly only near the end of exercise, it is critical to determine if the value immediately returns to normal as soon as exercise stops. An immediate normalization suggests that those abnormalities were spurious.

EXERCISE RECOVERY

Immediately after a maximal effort, subjects must maintain leg movement in recovery to support venous return. On a cycle ergometer, the pedaling resistance is turned off, and the subject is instructed to keep pedaling slowly. With treadmill exercise, the patient is instructed to step to the sides of the treadmill, off of the moving belt. Once the belt has stopped, the patient should step in place during the recovery.

Immediately after the test, the physician should ask the subject for the primary symptom that made them stop. The patient should specifically be queried about leg fatigue, dyspnea, chest pain, or lightheadedness, and that response should be recorded.

A normal individual at the end of a maximum CPET effort will usually describe leg fatigue as the primary limitation, with dyspnea as a secondary issue.

Gas exchange and ECG measurements are usually continued for three to five minutes after the maximal effort. The rate of decline of heart rate provides some measure of conditioning. Blood pressure should be checked at least twice early in recovery and should decline to near the resting values after five minutes. Recovery blood pressure measurement is especially important with unfit young subjects, who may develop vagally mediated hypotension and bradycardia after a full effort. With any suggestion of a vagal post-exercise response, the subject should be immediately moved to a supine posture and kept there until blood pressure returns to normal. For all subjects who have given a full effort, the respiratory R value will increase to values of 1.25–1.40 during exercise recovery, a manifestation of the very rapid post-exercise drop in oxygen consumption within the exercising muscle, contrasting with the much slower clearance of the more soluble carbon dioxide accumulated within the exercised muscles.

7

Interpreting the CPET

Following completion of the exercise test, two tasks remain. The first is to systematically evaluate all the data acquired. This step-by-step process will be illustrated using a normal data set that will also include a discussion of the range of normal responses for each measurement. The second and most important task is to translate those findings into a final report that is clinically meaningful for the health care provider requesting the test. It is important to remember that an overwhelming majority of medical professionals are not familiar with the measurements made during an exercise test, and the significance of abnormal findings need to be described with this recognition in mind. In addition, the patient being tested is obviously interested in the findings, and the summary of the report should be reader-friendly for a layperson.

EVALUATION OF THE DATA

Formatting the exercise data

Presentation of the breath-by-breath measurements made by modern exercise systems reveals a substantial amount of between-breath scatter for the measurements of oxygen consumption ($\dot{V}O_2$) and tidal volume (TV) (Figure 7.1).

Very little of this between-breath variability in $\dot{V}O_2$ reflects measurement error, but rather it represents the normal breath-by-breath variability in TV. Over 98% of the breath-by-breath variability in $\dot{V}O_2$ is accounted for by the variability in TV. As the increases in both $\dot{V}O_2$ and carbon dioxide output during a CPET progress smoothly at the muscle level, the breath-by-breath presentation of data is not helpful in the interpretation of the majority of clinical studies. Hence, the individual breath measurements of $\dot{V}O_2$ and $\dot{V}CO_2$ are summed in 20-second bins and expressed in terms of liters/minute. Minute ventilation ($\dot{V}E$) reflects the summed value of 20-second bins of TV measurements, expressed as liters/minute. The TV and heart-rate measurements on the data printout represent 20-second averages (Figure 7.2).

Maximal effort and maximal oxygen uptake

The primary measurement expected from a CPET is the maximal oxygen uptake ($\dot{V}O_2$ max). For a normal subject who has given a maximal exercise effort, the measurement represents the limit of oxygen transport from the air to the mitochondria of the working muscles. A maximal oxygen uptake measurement is reproducible over days within a 2%–3% range and is the variable that can be tracked in disease progression or regression, as well as in training states over longer periods of time. For nearly all exercise testing indications, it is important to be confident that the patient gave a maximal exercise effort, and in making that judgment, there are several observations to keep in mind.

First, the person conducting the test should have a good subjective sense of whether the exercise subject gave a full, symptom-limited effort. Supportive and enthusiastic coaching during the final minutes of the test is always important. Provided that the patient understands the rationale for giving a maximal effort, and understands the safety precautions in place during the test, it has been our experience that nearly everyone will give an acceptable and reproducible maximal effort. At the conclusion of the maximal effort it is helpful to have the patient identify their primary exercise-limiting symptom. For the majority of both normal subjects and subjects with cardiac impairment, the most common

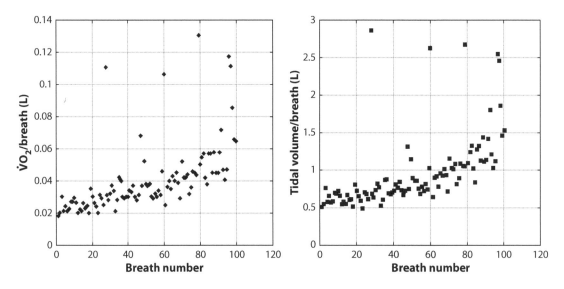

Figure 7.1 Per-breath measurements of oxygen consumption ($\dot{V}O_2$) and tidal volume (TV) during an early portion of a progressive work exercise test.

limiting symptom is leg fatigue, or the sense of sudden loss of leg power, with dyspnea as the limiting symptom for most of the others.

Second, if during the final stages of a maximal effort, both heart rate and oxygen uptake appear to plateau despite a progressively increasing ergometer work rate or treadmill grade, that finding strongly supports a truly maximal cardiac effort in a highly motivated subject. The maximal exercise heart rate achieved is not a useful indicator of a maximal effort unless it substantially exceeds an age-predicted normal value. Recall that among normal subjects of any age there is substantial variability in maximal exercise heart rate. In addition,

for patients with myocardial diseases, there is an almost universal reduction in maximal exercise heart rate.

The best objective criterion for a maximal cardiovascular effort is the identification of a ventilatory threshold (or "anaerobic threshold") at an appropriate time during the exercise effort. The ventilatory threshold is a marker for the onset of systemic washout of the local exercising muscle norepinephrine release and subsequent metabolic acidosis of heavy exercise. The threshold identification is ordinarily based on inspection of three CPET exhaled gas measurements. If arterial blood samples are acquired throughout a CPET, the

Time (sec)	$\dot{V}O_2$ (L/min)	$\dot{V}CO_2$ (L/min)	V_T (L)	HR (beats/min)
20	0.63	0.53	1.00	96
40	0.63	0.55	0.97	97
60	0.73	0.62	1.02	96
80	0.66	0.55	0.98	100
100	0.81	0.72	1.27	103
120	0.84	0.70	1.25	105
140	0.86	0.71	1.71	105
160	1.16	0.89	1.34	108
180	1.19	0.91	1.30	110
200	1.15	0.90	1.28	112
220	1.25	1.00	1.86	115
240	1.54	1.21	1.57	116

Figure 7.2 20-second averages of CPET measurements of oxygen consumption ($\dot{V}O_2$), carbon dioxide output ($\dot{V}CO_2$), tidal volume (V_T), and heart rate (HR) acquired at the early exercise stages of a typical test.

ventilatory threshold is best represented by the onset of the progressive rise in arterial blood lactate levels.

Identification and interpretation of the ventilatory threshold

The three approaches used to identify a ventilatory threshold from CPET data (V-slope, $\dot{V}E/\dot{V}O_2$, and end-tidal PO_2) were described in Chapter 5 (Figure 7.3).

It has been our practice to try to identify all three markers in determining a best single ventilatory threshold estimate. On average, a V-slope estimate will arise between 50% and 60% of a maximal CPET effort, and the two ventilation-based estimates ($\dot{V}E/\dot{V}O_2$ and end-tidal PO_2) arise between 60% and 70% of a maximal effort. The judgment of which estimate to weigh most heavily depends on the consistency of the measurements acquired during the particular study, but identification of a ventilatory threshold at an appropriate interval within a CPET represents the best marker for a maximal aerobic effort. The onset of a ventilatory threshold during a progressive work test is also associated with a more marked rise in systolic blood pressure, likely a consequence of the systemic washout of norepinephrine from nerve terminals in the exercising muscles.

While the normal range of values for onset of the ventilatory threshold described above is appropriate for young subjects, for older subjects, the threshold comes progressively later in a maximal performance, such that, in some apparently healthy 80-year-old subjects, the threshold may only arise in the final minute of a maximal effort. In addition, both muscle fiber type and training status influence the time of onset. Individuals who are (or had been) successful sprint or power athletes show relatively earlier ventilatory thresholds compared with individuals who could only succeed in endurance events. Endurance training, in addition to improving the maximal oxygen uptake, will also move the onset of the ventilatory threshold to a later point within a maximal CPET effort. Some fit aerobic endurance athletes with predominantly slow twitch muscle fiber types may not show a ventilatory threshold until they reach 90% of their $\dot{V}O_2$ max. Finally, for heart failure patients treated with high doses of beta blockers, the ventilatory threshold appears to come later in CPET efforts.

The respiratory R value ($\dot{V}CO_2/\dot{V}O_2$) increases progressively during an exercise test, first as a manifestation of the exercise shift from primary metabolism of fatty acids to carbohydrates, and finally to the washout of muscle CO_2 stores secondary to the hyperventilation response to the metabolic acidosis. While the time during an exercise study when the R exceeds 1.0 is usually close to the ventilatory threshold determined by any of the three criteria described above, the R value is also influenced by the CPET duration, anxiety, pretest dietary intake, training status, and other factors, so the CPET time when the R value exceeds 1.0 is not a reliable marker for identification of a ventilatory threshold. An R value of greater than 1.10 at maximal effort has been used in a number of studies to confirm that a maximal cardiovascular effort was expended, although many subjects will exceed that value for an additional two or three minutes during a test. However a well-trained endurance athlete giving an obvious maximal effort during a relatively prolonged progressive work test may not even reach an R value of 1.10.

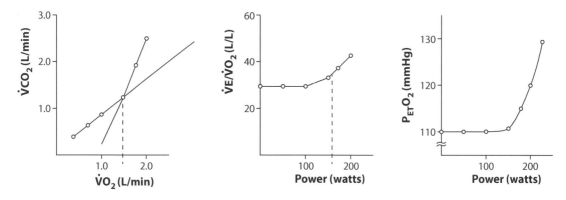

Figure 7.3 Ventilatory threshold identified by the V-slope approach (plot A), by increase in $\dot{V}E/\dot{V}O_2$ (plot B), and by increase in ETO_2 (plot C) during a progressive work test.

Normal predicted values

There are several different published data sets used to describe normal predicted values for maximal oxygen uptake that incorporate height, age, and sex as the inputs to calculate a predicted normal value. There are appreciable differences among these data sets describing predicted maximal oxygen uptake. For example, a 40-year-old male with a height of 180 cm will have a predicted maximal oxygen uptake of 3100 mL/min using the Jones data, based on "nonathletic" Canadians (Jones et al., 1985), 2900 mL/min using the Hansen data based on southern California industrial workers (Hansen et al., 1984), and 2500 mL/min using the Neder predictions utilizing a randomly selected group of clerical workers (Neder et al., 1999). The Jones predictions are more appropriate for active subjects, and the latter two are more appropriate for more sedentary subjects. An important reservation for all of these normal predicted values is that they use simple linear regression based on measurements from subjects between 20 and 70 years of age. Hence, the predicted values for young teenagers will be inappropriately high and predicted values for the normal elderly may be inappropriately low.

Sub-maximal exercise tests

Some studies have used measurements of oxygen consumption at a subject's age-predicted heart rate, or worse, oxygen consumption at 80% of a subject's age-predicted heart rate as a means of estimating maximal oxygen consumption. Because of the variability of age-predicted heart rate even in a normal population, both estimates have not been accurate for a given subject simply because of the large variability in estimated heart rate, an especially significant problem for older subjects. Other studies have stopped the exercise study once a ventilatory threshold has been identified. Because of the variable time of onset for a ventilatory threshold among individuals, assuming that the oxygen consumption at the ventilatory threshold can be used to estimate the maximal oxygen uptake again represents a poor estimate of that value. In summary, the maximal oxygen uptake is only reliably measured by maximal exercise test, and a properly conducted test is acceptably safe for nearly all patients with the relatively few exclusions described earlier.

Interpreting the maximal oxygen uptake measurement

As maximal oxygen uptake, similar to maximal cardiac output, is dependent on the subject's size, a universal convention has been to divide the maximal oxygen uptake (mL/min) by the subject's weight in kilograms (mL/kg/min). However, because of the prevalence of overweight or obese exercise subjects in current clinical practice, the maximal oxygen uptake should also be compared with a predicted value based on the subject's height, age, and sex, independent of weight. That latter comparison of maximal oxygen uptake as a percent of a predicted value for a normal-weight subject provides a better estimate of an obese subject's maximal cardiac output. However, the value of describing the $\dot{V}O_2$ max normalized by body weight in overweight and obese subjects is that it provides an estimate of the limitations they will face in activities of daily living due to their weight. In short, presenting $\dot{V}O_2$ max as a percent of a predicted value based on height, age, and sex is a surrogate representation of maximal cardiac pumping capacity, while $\dot{V}O_2$ max normalized by subject weight appropriately describes the functional capacity for a subject to engage in sustained activities such as uphill walking or running.

Cardiovascular response: ECG and heart rate

The ECG is recorded throughout the exercise test and recovery and should be constantly monitored for signs of ischemia or rhythm abnormalities. The heart rate during a CPET normally increases in a nearly linear fashion with increasing exercise demands, and any sudden change in heart rate during a CPET is strongly suggestive of the onset of an arrhythmia. Maximal exercise heart rate for a given individual is highly reproducible, but it is important to recall that, among normal individuals of the same age, there is appreciable variability in maximal exercise heart rate. Maximal exercise heart rate in general declines with age, although individuals who maintain a high level of physical activity show a slower decline. With those caveats, a rough estimate of predicted maximal heart rate is:

Predicted maximal exercise HR = 220 − age

For normal subjects, maximal exercise heart rate is modestly higher with treadmill exercise compared with ergometer exercise, but the difference is ordinarily less than 10 beats/minute. The relative contribution of exercise heart rate to maximal exercise capacity is obtained from calculation of *heart rate range*, the difference between a subject's resting heart rate and their maximal exercise heart rate. The resting cardiac output is constant among subjects of the same size, so that resting heart rate is inversely proportional to a subject's size-appropriate stroke volume. Thus a low resting heart rate reflects a larger body size-adjusted stroke volume. However the maximal exercise heart rate is not dependent on stroke volume, so that a relatively high maximal exercise heart rate is a second factor that increases the heart rate range and overall exercise cardiac output. The use of an age-predicted maximal heart rate to calculate a heart rate range is inappropriate because of the broad range of maximal exercise heart rates for subjects of the same age. Heart rate should also be recorded for three to five minutes of recovery, as a decline of less than 12 beats/minute one minute after exercise termination is a negative prognostic marker for cardiac patients. In contrast, a more rapid decrease in post-exercise heart rate is seen in aerobically fit subjects. However, for young unfit subjects who have given a maximal exercise effort, a rapidly dropping post-exercise heart rate, when associated with post-exercise hypotension, indicates an oncoming vagal reaction. Those subjects should be immediately helped to a supine position and kept there for several minutes.

Cardiovascular response: O_2 pulse

The O_2 pulse ($\dot{V}O_2$/HR) is a simple rearrangement of the Fick Equation. During a standard CPET, the changes in O_2 pulse reflect changes in two different exercise parameters: the stroke volume and the arterio-venous oxygen content difference.

$$O_2 \text{ pulse} = \dot{V}O_2/HR = SV \times (\text{Content arterial } O_2 \\ - \text{ Content mixed} \\ \text{venous } O_2)$$

Recall that, for normal subjects, once exercise leg movement begins, stroke volume increases and thereafter remains constant, whereas the difference between arterial oxygen content and mixed venous content increases linearly as the exercise intensity increases. Hence, for a normal subject, the O_2 pulse shows a small bump with initiation of exercise and increases steadily throughout the exercise effort (Figure 7.4).

Given that subjects with a wide range of exercise capacities will all attain mixed venous oxygen saturations of 25% or less with maximal effort, the absolute value of the O_2 pulse attained at maximal effort is a reasonable representation of stroke volume. Similar to stroke volume, the maximal O_2 pulse measurement is dependent on the subject size. However, it is important to recall that a maximal O_2 pulse value is also dependent on hemoglobin concentration and will necessarily be lower for subjects with anemia. On approaching maximal effort, the rate of increase in O_2 pulse may lessen slightly, possibly a consequence of a modest reduction in stroke volume with maximal heart rates. Nevertheless, a normal O_2 pulse measurement should always continue to increase with exercise intensity.

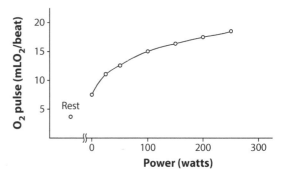

Figure 7.4 Plot of O_2 pulse throughout the course of a progressive work test.

Cardiovascular response: Blood pressure

The normal blood pressure response in a progressive work test shows little change between the resting and early exercise systolic pressures. With the onset of the systemic washout of norepinephrine and hydrogen ions from exercising muscle with heavy exercise, systolic pressure increases more rapidly, with final systolic pressures usually ranging between 150 and 200 mmHg with maximal effort. Patients with hypertension at rest may reach pressures of 230 mmHg. We have not used high systolic pressures as an indication to stop the test. The systolic pressure in recovery has usually returned to the resting range within two to three minutes. As noted in the discussion of exercise heart rate, the post-exercise blood pressure should be monitored, especially in unfit young subjects who have given a maximal effort, as they may manifest a hypotensive vagal response in the initial post-exercise minutes.

Pattern of exercise ventilation response

With a maximal effort, normal subjects ordinarily attain maximal exercise minute ventilation that is in the range of 60%–70% of their resting measurement of maximal voluntary ventilation. Another estimate of maximal ventilation capacity is obtained by multiplying the FEV_1 by 40. Ordinarily, both the $FEV_1 \times 40$ and the MVV estimates are quite close to each other, but when there is a discrepancy, it usually represents problems the subject had with the MVV maneuver, and the $FEV_1 \times 40$ estimate is the better choice. The difference between MVV or $FEV_1 \times 40$ and maximum exercise ventilation ($\dot{V}E$ max) is called the *ventilatory reserve*, representing the normal ventilation buffer between ventilation during a maximal exercise effort and the resting measurement of maximal ventilatory capacity (Figure 7.5). This ventilation buffer is lost or minimized in subjects with underlying pulmonary disorders.

The ventilation response to increasing effort during a standard CPET is linear until the final stages of exercise. In a normal subject, the slope of the linear portion of the $\dot{V}E$ vs. $\dot{V}CO_2$ graph is a reflection of the subject's overall ventilation sensitivity, and the constant slope reflects a constant exercise arterial $PaCO_2$. The point where the $\dot{V}E$ vs.

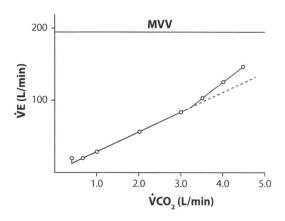

Figure 7.5 Normal pattern of increases in minute ventilation during a CPET plotted against exercise $\dot{V}CO_2$. The dashed line marks a continuation of the $\dot{V}E/\dot{V}CO_2$ slope measured in the early stages of exercise. The horizontal line represents the maximal voluntary ventilation measured at rest (MVV = 196 L/min).

$\dot{V}CO_2$ plot deviates from linearity during the CPET identifies the onset of the compensatory drop in $PaCO_2$ with heavy exercise. (Note that this point during a CPET comes *after* the ventilatory threshold.) In subjects with abnormal lungs and significant ventilation-perfusion mismatch, additional ventilation is required to maintain any given value of arterial CO_2, and hence the $\dot{V}E/\dot{V}CO_2$ slope will always be increased relative to what might be expected for the arterial $PaCO_2$. In addition, the $\dot{V}E/\dot{V}CO_2$ slope will be increased by any condition lowering arterial $PaCO_2$, such as metabolic acidosis or increased respiratory drive.

The exercise tidal volume response of a normal subject during a progressive work test is quite stereotypical. Tidal volume increases during exercise until it reaches roughly 60% of the vital capacity, and after that point, the ventilation increases by increases in respiratory rate alone. The work of breathing increases substantially for tidal volumes above 60% of the vital capacity, and for most subjects, additional increases in minute ventilation are achieved most efficiently by increases in respiratory rate. Some normal subjects will show a decrease in tidal volume at the very end of an exercise effort, associated with an extreme increase in respiratory rate (Figure 7.6).

Most computerized exercise systems now provide an option for the clinician to display and record the exercise flow-volume loops during

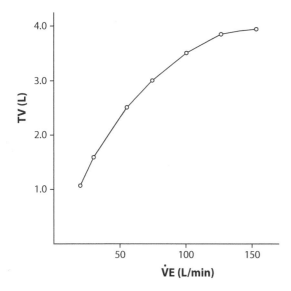

Figure 7.6 Progression of tidal volume plotted against minute ventilation for a normal subject during a CPET. (Vital capacity for this subject was 6.1 L.)

exercise. If exercise inspiratory capacity measurements have been acquired periodically through the test, the exercise tidal-volume loops can be superimposed on the maximal effort flow-volume loop measured before exercise. This option helps document whether there is expiratory (obstructive airway disease such as asthma or COPD) or inspiratory (upper airway or vocal cord dysfunction) flow limitation during exercise (Figure 7.7).

Ventilatory equivalents and ventilatory sensitivity

Ventilatory equivalents for O_2 and CO_2 reflect the amount of ventilation per liter of oxygen consumed or per liter of carbon dioxide exhaled. As noted in the discussion above on the ventilatory threshold, the point during exercise when the $\dot{V}E/\dot{V}O_2$ begins to increase is one marker for the onset of the metabolic acidosis of heavy exercise. (Note that the $\dot{V}E/\dot{V}O_2$ begins its consistent rise *after* the $\dot{V}E/\dot{V}O_2$ ventilatory threshold.) The values for these two ventilatory equivalent ratios before the onset of the ventilatory threshold are markers of ventilatory sensitivity in normal subjects. There is a wide range of normal exercise ventilatory sensitivity. Subjects with relatively low ventilatory equivalent values ($\dot{V}E/\dot{V}O_2$ values of 18–22 liters/liter) are

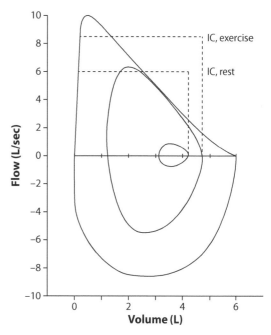

Figure 7.7 A resting flow-volume loop containing a loop representing resting breathing and a loop representing near maximal exercise. Inspiratory capacity (IC) during exercise is larger than IC at rest.

seen in subjects with relatively blunted ventilation response to exercise and hypoxia, and relatively high values ($\dot{V}E/\dot{V}O_2$ values of 29 to 32 liters/liter) are seen in subjects with a very brisk ventilation response to exercise and hypoxia (Figure 7.8).

While both ventilatory equivalent ratios provide an estimate of exercise ventilation sensitivity, the exercise $\dot{V}E/\dot{V}CO_2$ has been the more frequently

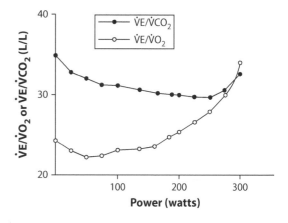

Figure 7.8 Stable values for both $\dot{V}E/\dot{V}O_2$ and $\dot{V}E/\dot{V}CO_2$ are attained in early and mid-exercise, before the onset of the ventilatory threshold.

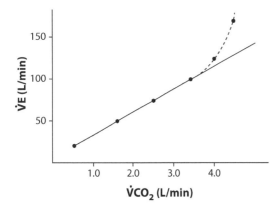

Figure 7.9 Measurement of $\dot{V}E/\dot{V}CO_2$ based on the slope of a straight line fit to the $\dot{V}E$ vs. $\dot{V}CO_2$ data prior to the ventilatory threshold.

cited index. For a subject with normal lungs and a relatively high resting arterial PCO_2, this is reflected during exercise by a low $\dot{V}E/\dot{V}CO_2$ and for a subject with a relatively low resting $PaCO_2$, by a relatively high $\dot{V}E/\dot{V}CO_2$ during exercise. A normal $\dot{V}E/\dot{V}CO_2$ measurement of sensitivity is derived from the slope of a $\dot{V}E$ vs. CO_2 plot up to the CO_2 ventilatory threshold. Normal values encompass a large range, from 22 liters/liter CO_2 to 33 liters/liter CO_2 (Figure 7.9).

Exercise gas exchange

All CPETs include continuous monitoring of arterial oxygen saturation.

Normal subjects will not demonstrate arterial desaturation during a progressive work protocol test. However, particularly when oximeter finger probes are used during heavy exercise, reductions in oxygen saturation frequently arise, but are never confirmed if simultaneous arterial blood gas measurements are obtained. While a desaturation measurement artifact is less of a problem with forehead oximetry probes, desaturation artifacts during maximal exercise still happen. From exercise studies done on patients with known intrapulmonary shunts, however, a very useful pattern of true desaturation is noted. First, the level of desaturation will increase progressively as the workload increases, an effect due to the progressive exercise-induced desaturation in mixed venous blood entering the lungs. Second, in the minute immediately following the cessation of exercise, the true desaturation will persist or even increase for 30–60 seconds before resolving during exercise recovery. With a saturation motion artifact,

a reduction in saturation corrects almost immediately when the subject is no longer fighting to crank the pedals or keep up with the treadmill.

End-tidal CO_2 and arterial CO_2 measurements are nearly identical at rest in normal subjects, but with heavy exercise, the end-tidal CO_2 exceeds the arterial measurement, increasing to as much as 6 mmHg higher than arterial values with maximal effort. This happens because, during heavy exercise within a single breath, at the end of inspiration, the alveolar CO_2 is below the average arterial CO_2, and at end exhalation, it is above the mean arterial PCO_2. Hence while *mean* alveolar PCO_2 is quite close to arterial PCO_2 throughout exercise, a normal subject will show a slow increase in end-tidal CO_2 during moderately heavy exercise that only begins to decrease with the extreme ventilation of a maximal effort.

If arterial blood gas measurements have been obtained during exercise, the physiologic dead space can be calculated using the mixed expired CO_2 value (P_ECO_2) calculated from the CPET $\dot{V}E$ and $\dot{V}CO_2$ measurements taken at the time of the blood draw:

$$P_ECO_2 = 863 \times \dot{V}CO_2/\dot{V}E$$

$$V_D/V_T = (PaCO_2 - P_ECO_2)/PaCO_2$$

For a normal subject undergoing a CPET, a physiologic dead space measurement will progressively decrease from between 30% and 40% at rest to less than 20% with maximal effort. (Note that the V_D/V_T calculation presented by the software in some exercise testing systems uses the end-tidal PCO_2 measurement in place of the arterial measurement, yielding a calculated physiologic dead space that is higher than the correct value.)

In addition, with exercise arterial blood gases, the alveolar-arterial O_2 difference ($[A\text{-}a]DO_2$) can be calculated using the blood gas PaO_2 and $PaCO_2$ along with the R value measured at the time of the arterial blood draw.

$$PAO_2 = 150 - (PaCO_2/R)$$

$$(A\text{-}a)DO_2 = PAO_2 - PaO_2$$

In normal subjects during exercise, the difference is less than 10 mmHg until near maximal effort is approached, when it may increase to as much as 20 mmHg.

THE EXERCISE REPORT

The exercise report must communicate the findings to a number of people who are interested in the results. Hence, it must be useful for the referring physician, the patient, and other interested persons who the patient might select. In that light, the interpretation of the CPET must not only be "numbers" but also represent an interpretation of those measurements relative to the symptoms and performance limitations the patient has described.

A suggested format for that report:

1. Patient identification and clinical question posed
2. Exercise-relevant history
3. Exercise protocol and measurements taken
4. Exercise duration, limiting symptoms, and patient effort
5. Aerobic capacity ($\dot{V}O_2$ max) as % predicted and as expected from history and ventilatory threshold
6. Cardiac response
7. Ventilation response
8. Gas exchange response
9. Impression

Patient identification

Include age, gender, referral source, occupation, and the clinical question posed requiring the exercise test.

Exercise-relevant history

This section should include a description of the patient's exercise baseline prior to the development of symptoms. Either occupational exercise requirements or recreational or athletic accomplishments are all helpful. The duration and progression of the exercise symptoms, specifically as they impair the patient's occupational performance, sports performance, and/or activities of daily living should be documented. Finally, the previous exercise-relevant medications, medical evaluations, and tests should be summarized.

Exercise protocol and measurements

This section should describe the progressive work test as an exercise test continuing to a symptom-limited maximal effort with a total testing time of roughly 20 minutes. A description of the exercise device chosen and the rationale for choice of that device should be described. (An accurate description of the chosen exercise protocol is important as a point of reference for comparison with future tests.) A precise account of the format of the protocol should be explained (e.g., pace of increment of the treadmill's speed and incline or the progressive increase per minute of the workload on the cycle ergometer).

Document that you have explained the risks and rationale for performing the test to the patient and acquired signed informed consent to perform the study. Preparation of the patient includes performance of spirometry with flow-volume loops before the exercise test, followed by placement of 12-lead ECG, placement of oximeter or arterial line, and facemask or mouthpiece, and all are documented.

Describe the measurements acquired during and after the test, including continuous ECG recording, regular measurements of blood pressure, continuous measurement of ventilation volume, oxygen consumption, carbon dioxide output, oxygen saturation measurements, and (if obtained) blood gases.

Exercise duration, symptoms, and effort

Describe the total exercise time, maximal exercise level attained, subjective exercise-limiting symptoms described by the patient, and your impression of whether the patient gave a maximal effort. Also describe whether the patient felt the limiting symptoms at the end of the test reproduced what they ordinarily experience when they attempt heavy exercise.

Aerobic capacity

Describe the maximal oxygen uptake both in mL/kg/min and as a percent of a predicted value for the patient. Describe whether or not the predicted value chosen would have been appropriate to the patient in their presymptomatic condition, and whether the current measurement represents a measurement that is consistent with the patient's description of exercise limitation. Assuming a ventilatory threshold was identified during the exercise effort, describe how this measurement provides evidence for a maximal cardiac effort as the primary exercise limitation. Describe how maximal oxygen uptake is ordinarily determined by the maximal possible oxygen delivery to the exercising muscles, provided that there were no other limitations such as ventilation abnormalities, oxygen desaturation during exercise, or joint pain.

Cardiac response

Describe any ECG abnormalities noted during or after the test, and whether rhythm abnormalities or ischemic changes could contribute to the symptoms described. Describe the blood pressure responses to initial and final stages of exercise and to post-exercise recovery. Describe the maximal exercise heart rate observed, with appropriate caveats about age-predicted maximal heart rates if the value was relatively low. If the maximal O_2 pulse was low or failed to show a normal increase during the test, describe how this is an indirect estimate of stroke volume and that a failure to increase during later phases of the test suggests an abnormal progressive loss of stroke volume at higher exercise heart rates.

Ventilation response

Describe the resting spirometry results and compare the resting maximal voluntary ventilation with the maximal exercise ventilation and calculate the ventilatory reserve. Describe whether obstruction to airflow measured by spirometry was present and whether or not tidal volume decreased as respiratory rate increased. If exercise inspiratory capacity measurements were obtained, describe resting and exercise flow/volume loops to see if there was airflow limitation on exhalation (e.g., asthma or COPD) or on inhalation (e.g., variable upper airway dysfunction) or on both (e.g., fixed airway obstruction).

Also, describe whether or not there was a decrease in end-tidal CO_2 near the end of the test to document the absence (or presence) of a ventilation limitation to exercise. If the $\dot{V}E/\dot{V}CO_2$ was elevated, describe how this abnormality can be due to either an abnormally increased drive to breathe and/or primary lung abnormalities.

Gas exchange

Describe oxygen saturation measurements during exercise. If blood gas measurements were obtained, describe how the physiologic dead space and alveolar-arterial O_2 difference calculations changed throughout the test. (Making these calculations is often an option within an exercise system's software once the appropriate arterial blood gas measurements are available.) Describe how any abnormalities observed would assist in the diagnostic process.

Impression

A well-written succinct impression of the entire test is critical to communicate to both physician and patient the salient features of the test. The final impression should identify whether the exercise response was within the expected normal range for that individual or whether the findings suggest a pattern of cardiac, ventilatory, or pulmonary vascular/interstitial lung disease abnormalities. A synthesis of the pattern observed and how that might relate to the symptoms and findings that led to the request for the test should be summarized.

REFERENCES

Jones NL, Makrides L, Hitchcock C, Chypchar T, McCartney N. 1985. Normal standards for an incremental progressive cycle ergometer test. *Am Rev Resp Dis*, 131(5):700–708.

Hansen JE, Sue DY, Wasserman K. 1984. Predicted values for clinical exercise testing. *Am Rev Resp Dis*, 129:Suppl S49–S55.

Neder JA, Nery LE, Castelo A, Andreoni S, Lerario MC, Sachs A, Silva AC, Whipp BJ. 1999. Prediction of metabolic and cardiopulmonary responses to maximum cycle ergometry: A randomised study. *Eur Resp J*, 14:1304–1313.

8

Exercise testing patients with cardiovascular disease

The first extensively applied clinical exercise test used 12-lead ECG measurements acquired during and after a progressive work treadmill test. Although isolated exercise ECG studies are now requested less frequently, the ECG exercise data remain an important component of a full cardiopulmonary exercise test. For patients with advanced heart failure or adult congenital heart disease, full cardiopulmonary exercise tests provide essential prognostic information to guide treatment options, and CPET studies performed for that indication constitute a major portion of the consultation load for some exercise laboratories.

This chapter discusses the following:

- Diagnostic exercise electrocardiography
- Exercise-associated rhythm abnormalities
- Patterns of cardiac response in heart failure patients
- Patterns of ventilation response in heart failure patients
- Risk stratification based on CPET findings
- Exercise-associated autonomic abnormalities

The application of progressive work exercise protocols to clinical cardiology practice began almost 60 years ago. The goal of the original exercise ECG test was to determine whether a maximal exercise effort would reveal evidence for cardiac ischemia in patients who had a normal resting ECG. The clinical protocol involved recording a standard 12-lead ECG throughout a progressive exercise treadmill protocol to a symptom-limited maximal effort and a five-minute post-exercise recovery period. Although the original exercise ECG application to detect ischemic heart disease is now often supplanted by more sensitive and specific exercise ultrasound or exercise nuclear medicine tests, monitoring for exercise duration, arrhythmia, or exercise ECG evidence of cardiac ischemia remain essential safety components of any maximal exercise test. Diagnostic cardiopulmonary exercise tests to evaluate causes of dyspnea for patients who do not have typical angina symptoms may reveal ECG signs of cardiac ischemia, especially for patients who have atypical symptomatic presentations for coronary ischemia.

The ECG criterion for exercise-induced ischemia with the best balance between sensitivity and specificity is the development of at least a 1-mm horizontal or downsloping ST segment during or after exercise and persistence of that depression during the exercise recovery period (Figure 8.1).

For a patient demonstrating ischemic changes, the depth of the ST segment depression achieved, the number of involved leads, and the duration of those abnormalities during recovery all suggest more significant coronary stenosis. In addition to exercise-associated ST depression in the lateral chest leads, other important abnormalities associated with cardiac ischemia include development of ST elevation in lead aVR and development of bundle branch block during exercise. In current practice, a diagnostic CPET revealing ECG evidence of unexpected and untreated coronary ischemia does not necessarily require completion of the test to a maximal effort if the ECG changes suggest severe coronary stenosis. For any newly detected exercise ischemic abnormality,

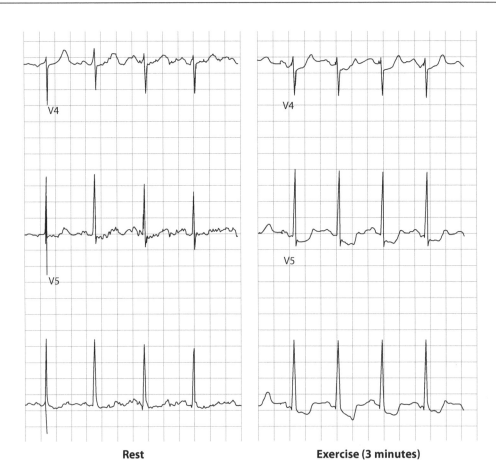

Rest   **Exercise (3 minutes)**

Figure 8.1 Development of 2-mm horizontal ST depression during an early stage of exercise.

confirmatory testing utilizing exercise echocardiography or exercise nuclear medicine images provide more sensitive and specific information concerning the anatomy of the ischemic abnormality.

The original exercise ECG studies also measured oxygen consumption during the treadmill exercise protocol and described an excellent correlation between maximal oxygen consumption achieved (described as mL O_2/kg/minute) and total treadmill time. While the subsequent clinical application of treadmill exercise ECG studies did not include measurements of oxygen consumption, the total exercise treadmill time attained by a patient still provides a reasonable estimate of maximal oxygen uptake if the patient is not overweight or obese. In the terminology of the original exercise ECG test, that maximal oxygen uptake estimate based on duration of the treadmill test was described as a percentage of the predicted normal value, termed the "functional aerobic impairment," in which a positive value represented a below-normal maximal oxygen uptake.

EXERCISE RHYTHM ABNORMALITIES

In the early era of diagnostic ECG treadmill testing, patients with untreated cardiac ischemia frequently developed multifocal premature ventricular beats, runs of ventricular tachycardia, and occasional cardiac arrest. The quoted risk from that era was one death in 10,000 exercise tests. In our current era, referred cardiac patients have undergone appropriate medical management before being sent for testing, and thus the risks of performing a maximal work exercise test are substantially lower than they were in the earlier era of cardiac exercise testing. In higher risk patients with heart failure and reduced ejection fraction, treatment with beta blockers and defibrillators has very appreciably reduced the incidence of serious arrhythmias and mortality during or after maximal exercise testing. Although the risk for cardiac arrest during or after a maximal exercise test will never be zero, even for those high-risk patients who have experienced appropriate defibrillator shocks at home, a shock during or after an exercise test is a very uncommon event. The primary ventricular arrhythmia risk during a diagnostic CPET today arises with patients sent for diagnostic testing when cardiac disease was not suspected. All patients undergoing a CPET should have their exercise and post-exercise rhythm monitored continuously, as it is very easy to miss two- or three-beat runs of ventricular tachycardia. Patients who show increasing frequency of ventricular premature contractions, including multifocal VPCS or bigeminy with increasing exercise effort are not normal, and the exercise effort should be terminated with appropriate cool-down measures described for abnormal blood pressure responses. In that immediate recovery period, the arrhythmias may be more frequent than they were during the exercise portion of the test. Finally, it is important to recall that unifocal ventricular premature contractions that are noted at rest and during early exercise, but that disappear as the exercise load increases, are a relatively common finding and are benign.

Supraventricular rhythm abnormalities can also develop during or after an exercise test. Atrial fibrillation developing during sustained heavy exercise is a relatively common finding in some active elderly patients who have noted an episodic reduction in their exercise capacity. If their blood pressure response remains appropriate for the level of exercise, the test can continue to a maximal effort. However regular supraventricular tachycardias are not well tolerated and require removal of the exercise load, as these arrhythmias often persist into the recovery period and may require additional diagnosis and treatment. As described above for patients with significant ventricular ectopy, the exercise load should be removed, and the patients should continue to move their legs to maintain venous return during the initial cool down period. They should be monitored with blood pressure and ECG measurements until the supraventricular tachycardia is resolved.

Because most myocardial diseases manifest some degree of chronotropic limitation during exercise, using attainment of an age-predicted maximal heart rate as an indicator of maximal effort is especially inappropriate for patients with cardiac disease. With the exception of patients with isolated valvular heart disease or patients with surgically corrected congenital heart disease, most patients with cardiac abnormalities are not able to attain normal age-predicted maximal exercise heart rates. In addition, a majority of patients with ischemic disease and/or heart failure are treated with beta blockers. Once a patient has been maintained on a given dose of beta blocker for several weeks, the maximal oxygen uptake is only minimally reduced, despite some very appreciable reductions in maximal exercise heart rate. The mechanism responsible for the increased exercise stroke volume that develops with this treatment is not clear, but the effect is a consistent one. For patients treated with beta blockers, the appearance of a ventilatory threshold at about 65%–80% of a maximal effort remains the best available marker for a maximal effort in these patients with a pharmacological reduction in maximal chronotropic response. With the intense beta blockade administered to the most severely impaired heart failure patients, it often is more difficult to identify a clear ventilatory threshold, but for these patients, the V-slope method is most helpful.

THE CARDIOVASCULAR PATTERN OF RESPONSE IN HEART FAILURE

The overall pattern of CPET response for a patient with mild or moderate heart failure may only differ from the exercise pattern of a normal subject by a relative reduction in maximal oxygen consumption. In common with normal subjects, heart failure patients undergoing a CPET will demonstrate a ventilatory threshold and progressive increase in blood pressure at roughly 65%–80% of the duration of a progressive work test to maximal effort. In addition, as with normal subjects, patients with heart failure giving a maximal effort in a progressive work test will extract 70%–75% of the oxygen from arterial blood during a maximal CPET effort, so that the difference in maximal oxygen uptake between normal subjects and heart failure subjects is attributable to a lower cardiac output alone. Given the substantial range of maximal oxygen uptakes among normal subjects, a modest reduction in maximal oxygen consumption is difficult to prove as abnormal unless the subject had undergone an exercise test before the onset of new exercise symptoms. A rough estimate of a patient's prior exercise tolerance can usually be made with physically active patients, but exercise history is less helpful for subjects who have been resolutely sedentary prior the development of their new symptoms.

An exercise report of maximal oxygen uptake reports the measurement normalized by the subject's weight (mL O_2/kg/min), an adjustment for different body size based on the obvious fact that big people will consume more oxygen than small people. However, normalizing maximal oxygen consumption by weight can be misleading with respect to cardiac risk. Recall that the maximal oxygen uptake is valued as the best noninvasive surrogate measurement of maximal cardiac output. However, the decision to normalize the measurement by the subject's weight will lead to deceptively low numbers for obese patients. If the purpose of an exercise test were to estimate the walking or running pace that an obese patient could sustain, then weight normalization does make sense, as that adjusts for the higher energy expenditure required to move a large body. However, for a cardiac patient, the goal of the test is to obtain an estimate of the maximal cardiac output, regardless of the patient's BMI, so that maximal oxygen consumption described as a percent of a predicted value for maximal oxygen uptake that is based on a patient's height, age, and sex represents the more appropriate choice. Unfortunately, even in our age of epidemic obesity, the cardiology literature may describe only weight-normalized $\dot{V}O_2$ max measurements. Because of that convention, the severity of cardiac impairment of the occasional heart failure patient with a very low BMI whose $\dot{V}O_2$ impairment is described in mL/kg/min will be substantially underestimated.

THE O_2 PULSE AS A MARKER FOR FORWARD STROKE VOLUME

Recall that normal subjects maintain a relatively constant stroke volume after the initiation of upright leg exercise and that, with a maximal sustained exercise effort, both normal subjects and cardiac patients can extract roughly 75% of the arterial oxygen content when the mixed venous blood returns to the heart. Because a maximal cardiovascular effort yields the same magnitude of arterio-venous oxygen extraction in patients with and without heart disease, the Fick equation

shows that the difference in oxygen consumption for same-sized patients with and without heart disease is due to differences in cardiac output alone.

$$\text{Fick equation: } \dot{V}O_2 = \text{Cardiac output} \times \\ \text{(Arterio-venous } O_2 \\ \text{difference)}$$

As cardiac output is simply the product of the heart rate and stroke volume, the O_2 pulse calculation during exercise will rise progressively, in parallel with the progressive increase in arterio-venous O_2 extraction.

$$O_2 \text{ pulse equation: } \dot{V}O_2/HR = \text{Stroke volume} \times \\ \text{(Arterio-venous} \\ O_2 \text{ difference)}$$

Hence, the O_2 pulse measurement at maximal effort represents a noninvasive estimate that correlates well with stroke volume for both normal subjects and cardiac patients. Decreased values are expected for patients with cardiac impairment at maximal effort. It is important to remember that the maximal O_2 pulse as a stroke volume estimate is dependent on both subject size (because it includes $\dot{V}O_2$) and hemoglobin concentration (because that is another determinant of the arterial-mixed venous oxygen content difference).

For patients with cardiac disease, the course of O_2 pulse measurement during exercise can provide additional insight into their impaired ventricular function. In a normal subject, a normal O_2 pulse response increases steadily during the test, sometimes tending toward a plateau in the final minute or two of testing. However, for patients with a significant component of diastolic dysfunction or any other cause of exercise-associated reduction in stroke volume, the O_2 pulse will fail to increase despite the progressive increases in oxygen consumption (Figure 8.2).

For patients with heart failure and preserved ejection fraction as the cause of exercise limitation, left ventricular filling is impaired as the heart rate increases, so stroke volume decreases concurrent with the normal increase in O_2 extraction from mixed venous blood. The net effect is flattening or even a decrease in O_2 pulse as exercise progresses. As the initial stages of diastolic dysfunction may not be apparent on resting echocardiography, an abnormal progression of O_2 pulse can represent the first information suggesting the presence of

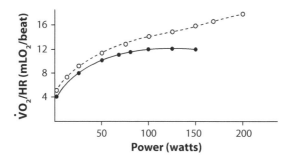

Figure 8.2 O_2 pulse measurements during a CPET for a normal subject (open circles) and for a subject with significant diastolic dysfunction (closed circles).

exercise impairment from diastolic dysfunction. Although diastolic dysfunction is the most common cause of an abnormal O_2 pulse profile, valvular heart disease, severe pulmonary hypertension, or exercise-induced atrial fibrillation may also produce an abnormal O_2 pulse profile during the final stages of a test. Whatever the responsible mechanism, an O_2 pulse that fails to increase during the final third of a full exercise effort is an abnormality that indicates a loss of forward stroke volume at higher heart rates.

EXERCISE BLOOD PRESSURE ABNORMALITIES

The essential safety insight gained from the initial era of exercise ECG testing for coronary artery disease was the importance of monitoring exercise blood pressure. Normal subjects show modest increases in systolic blood pressure during the initial phases of an exercise test and show much more substantial increases in systolic pressure with the onset of exercise-associated acidosis. Cardiac patients who fail to increase their blood pressure during heavy exertion are at high risk for ventricular arrhythmias during or immediately following a maximal exercise effort. Any patient who decreases or fails to appropriately increase systolic blood pressure during heavy exertion should have their exercise load withdrawn. This exercise precaution is especially relevant for patients with severe ischemic heart disease, idiopathic cardiomyopathy, hypertrophic cardiomyopathy, aortic stenosis, or severe pulmonary hypertension. During exercise recovery, these high-risk patients must be encouraged to continue leg movement with unloaded pedaling or stepping to support venous return to the heart and receive sustained post-exercise monitoring of blood pressure and heart rhythm. This abnormal blood pressure response to exercise merits prompt clinical follow-up to determine if additional treatment options are available.

EXERCISE VENTILATION ABNORMALITIES IN CHRONIC HEART FAILURE

While the exercise ventilation pattern of patients with mild heart failure cannot be distinguished from a normal subject, some consistent exercise ventilation abnormalities become more apparent with more severe heart failure. For any level of oxygen consumption or CO_2 output during exercise, patients with symptomatic heart failure demonstrate an increased ventilation response throughout exercise (Figure 8.3).

Normal subjects will have a $\dot{V}E/\dot{V}CO_2$ slope (measured prior to the ventilatory threshold) in

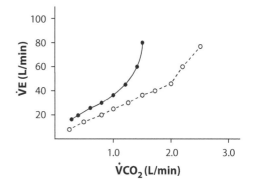

Figure 8.3 $\dot{V}E$ vs. $\dot{V}CO_2$ for normal subject (open circles) and an HF patient (closed circles)—note the augmented exercise ventilation response in the heart failure patient.

the 22–32 liters/liter range, while higher values are present in symptomatic heart failure patients. This increased ventilation response with exercise is associated with increased exercising muscle sympathetic nerve activity and carotid sinus sensitization to the elevated levels of angiotensin and catecholamines observed in chronic heart failure. The carotid sinus sensitization of heart failure patients is also revealed by their increased ventilation response to even the modest levels of hypoxia experienced at altitudes of 1500 meters.

Another abnormality in the ventilation response to exercise seen in the most severely impaired heart failure patients is a Cheyne–Stokes breathing pattern. This striking periodic variation in tidal volume produces regular oscillations in all of the measurements made at the mouth. However, the regular character of these variations is not obvious when the respiratory data are averaged in 20-second blocks, a presentation option that effectively conceals the sinusoidal-appearing breathing pattern. This exercise abnormality cannot be reliably identified without the capacity to present the respiratory measurements in a breath-by-breath format, as illustrated below (Figure 8.4).

To differentiate this periodic breathing pattern from an anxious patient with a simple irregular breathing response in early exercise, the breath-by-breath sinusoidal shifts during exercise should have a complete cycle length of 60–90 seconds, and at least three cycles should be apparent beginning with the onset of exercise. The sinusoidal pattern usually disappears near maximal effort. It is important to be aware of this abnormality, as it is easily missed if only the 20-second average data are examined.

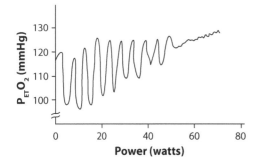

Figure 8.4 Periodic breathing in a patient with severe heart failure during exercise, illustrated by regular variation in end-tidal PO_2 measurements.

Patients with stable symptomatic heart failure demonstrate modest reductions in lung volumes and diffusing capacity, and these abnormalities persist even after aggressive diuresis. That decrease in diffusing capacity could represent modest increases in alveolar-capillary membrane thickness and/or varying amounts of extra-vascular lung water. Although heart failure patients with otherwise normal lungs do not demonstrate any signs suggestive of ventilatory limitation during exercise, they do show a relative reduction in maximal exercise tidal volume. Normal subjects will utilize about 60% of their vital capacity for ventilation during heavy exercise, while heart failure patients may only reach maximal exercise tidal volumes of 40% or 50% of their vital capacity. This heart failure exercise ventilation pattern may be attributable to decreased lung compliance or to the heart failure-associated increase in carotid body sensitivity. Whatever the mechanism, a relatively smaller exercise tidal volume with heavy exercise is a common finding in patients with significant heart failure.

CPET FOR RISK STRATIFICATION OF HEART FAILURE PATIENTS

Echocardiography is an essential tool in cardiology diagnosis, but has proven less useful for assessment of risk of death in heart failure patients. Direct measurement of maximal oxygen uptake provides the best noninvasive index of forward cardiac output and is a far stronger predictor of risk of cardiac death than a reduced ejection fraction. While echocardiographic measurement of ejection fraction (EF) remains the defining index of systolic heart failure, it is a relatively weak tool for risk assessment in comparison to measurement of maximal oxygen consumption. Even among patients selected for an EF of less than 25%, the range of exercise tolerance can be very wide, ranging from a patient still able to play doubles tennis to a patient with heart failure symptoms at rest. In contrast to the very strong relationship between maximal oxygen uptake and maximum cardiac output, the relationship between EF and maximal oxygen uptake is weak, and the reasons for the poor predictive value of EF for maximal cardiac output arises from several different sources. A variable degree of diastolic dysfunction accompanies most myocardial diseases, and that abnormality is not reflected by the EF. The echocardiographic indices suggesting the presence of diastolic dysfunction are less quantitative and are not always carefully evaluated in echocardiographic reports. Secondly, the EF, although a very reproducible measurement, is a ratio and hence does not represent the stroke volume. For a given value of EF, a large dilated heart will have a larger stroke volume in comparison to a less abnormal appearing heart that has the same EF. Finally, in addition to diastolic dysfunction, concomitant coronary ischemia, hypervolemia, valvular abnormalities, or pulmonary hypertension will all reduce maximal exercise cardiac output independent of a resting ejection fraction measurement.

For patients diagnosed with ischemic or idiopathic heart failure who are stable on optimal medical treatment, the primary indication for a CPET is to follow a measurement of maximal oxygen uptake for risk assessment. As patients with heart failure maintain the normal capacity to maximally extract oxygen from arterial blood during a maximal exercise effort, the measurement of maximal oxygen uptake is a direct reflection of the maximal cardiac output for these patients, just as it is for normal subjects. For most centers treating patients with advanced heart failure, a $\dot{V}O_2$ max of less that 12–14 mL/kg/min in a clinically stabilized patient is a quantitative marker of advanced disease and high risk for death, prompting consideration of transplant listing or insertion of a left ventricular assist device.

The $\dot{V}E/\dot{V}CO_2$ slope measurement has additional prognostic predictive power for heart failure patients, independent of the $\dot{V}O_2$ max measurement. The original risk assessment used only the initial portion of the $\dot{V}E$ vs. $\dot{V}CO_2$ plot, ignoring the final extreme hyperventilation at maximal effort. However, the slope of a line fit all of the breath-by-breath measurements on a $\dot{V}E$ vs. $\dot{V}CO_2$ exercise plot has proven to provide a superior risk assessment for heart failure patients (Figure 8.5).

As patients with severe heart failure tend to show extreme hyperventilation with maximal effort, applying a linear fit to all of the exercise data produces a steeper slope than the traditional fit that only includes measurements up to the ventilatory threshold. For heart failure patients, risk of cardiac death increases if the measured slope is in the 35–39 liters/liter range, with a yet greater risk for a slope in the 40–44 range, and the highest

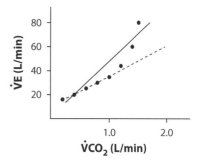

Figure 8.5 The $\dot{V}E/\dot{V}CO_2$ slope fit used for evaluation of heart failure patients (solid line) compared with the fit traditionally used to evaluate exercise ventilation (dashed line).

risk for values above 45 liters/liter CO_2. This measurement abnormality also has adverse predictive power for heart failure patients even if their $\dot{V}O_2$ max is better than 20 mL/kg/min.

A third, more recently accepted exercise ventilation risk factor relevant for the most severely impaired heart failure patients is the Cheyne–Stokes breathing pattern described above. Patients presenting with this periodic breathing abnormality during exercise have the same prognosis as a patient with New York Heart Association class IV symptoms. The exercise prognostic finding adds to risk assessment from the $\dot{V}O_2$ max measurement and is helpful if the periodic breathing persists throughout the CPET, making an appropriate estimate of the $\dot{V}E/\dot{V}CO_2$ slope challenging.

AUTONOMIC EXERCISE ABNORMALITY: THE POTS SYNDROME

The autonomic regulation of blood pressure and flow during exercise is essential for even modest levels of exertion. The balance of demand for blood flow from large exercising muscle beds and the requirement for adequate pressure for both cerebral and coronary perfusion represents a complex regulatory response whose mechanisms are incompletely understood. The postural orthostasis tachycardia syndrome (POTS) represents a poorly understood malady in which this balance is lost. The clinical presentation of this syndrome is similar to dysautonomia. Lightheadedness, near syncope, palpitations, and fatigue are present and are usually brought on by exertion or orthostatic changes. These previously exercise-normal patients are predominantly younger women (females > males; 5:1) who have no evidence of myocardial abnormalities. They may present suddenly with symptoms of a decrease in exercise tolerance that is apparent as they approach half of their prior maximal exercise capacity. Previously healthy aerobic athletes suddenly become consistently symptomatic and cannot continue training. Unfortunately, these patients often remain symptomatic for a sustained period of time before their diagnosis is recognized.

The diagnosis is often identified during a CPET. The hallmark of POTS during a progressive work test is a normal chronotropic response, but a failure to increase blood pressure at moderate to high levels of exertion or even a drop in blood pressure at these levels. Confirmatory testing includes tilt table tests and other autonomic measurements, although echocardiograms and cortisol and catecholamine levels should be considered to rule out other etiologies. Although the diagnosis of POTS is not difficult if suspected, the spectrum of overlapping etiologies is broad. Thus, treatment may require trials of various medications best managed by physicians who are familiar with the syndrome. For example, fludrocortisone, salt loading, SSRI, and beta-blockers have been helpful, each by a different mechanism of action, hinting at the multiple etiologies that may trigger the clinical presentation. Low-level exercise training appears to provide some benefit during recovery. Patients with severe symptoms are very limited; others with moderate or mild symptoms may continue to be active on a cautious level. The syndrome may spontaneously abate over months or may persist and require trials of various treatments.

SUMMARY POINTS

- Maximal oxygen uptake is a robust surrogate estimate of maximum cardiac output for heart failure patients as well as for normal subjects.
- As with normal subjects, patients with cardiac impairment giving a maximal exercise effort will manifest a ventilatory threshold at roughly 65%–75% of a maximal effort, although they are unlikely to reach a normal age-predicted maximal heart rate.
- Heart failure patients have an increased ventilatory response to exercise, with an increased $\dot{V}E/\dot{V}CO_2$ slope and a ventilation pattern of increased respiratory rate with reduced exercise tidal volume.
- CPET testing of patients with severe heart failure provides the best ability to guide advanced treatment options, using both changes in $\dot{V}O_2$ max and the $\dot{V}E/\dot{V}CO_2$ slope for decision points.
- Exercise electrocardiography for diagnosis of ischemic heart disease has been supplanted by cardiac exercise echo, but exercise electrocardiography can reveal unexpected ischemic heart disease and remains an essential element of exercise test safety.
- The pattern of response of the O_2 pulse during a progressive work test provides insight into the potential presence of diastolic dysfunction as a limiting component for a patient with exercise limitation.
- The postural orthostasis tachycardia syndrome (POTS) impairs exercise capacity despite normal myocardial function because of abnormal exercise-associated autonomic responses.

9

Exercise testing patients with pulmonary hypertension

The right and left ventricles ordinarily move the same volume of blood with each beat but operate under quantitatively different hemodynamics. The normal pulmonary vasculature is a low-resistance system with a mean arterial pressure of around 15 mmHg at rest that only increases to the range of 20–25 mmHg with a five-fold or more increase in cardiac output. Compared with the systemic vasculature, the pulmonary vascular tree is a very compliant and recruitable vascular network. However, a number of diseases involving the pulmonary vasculature cause dramatic losses of that pulmonary vascular compliance, resulting in higher pulmonary artery pressures with rest and exercise. When pulmonary vascular disease increases that resistance, the right ventricle cannot fully compensate for the increased pulmonary vascular pressures, particularly with the added demands of exercise, and cardiac output is limited. This chapter describes the following:

- Classification of etiologies of pulmonary hypertension
- Clinical presentation of patients with pulmonary artery hypertension (PAH)
- Pattern of CPET response for PAH patients
- Exercise gas exchange abnormalities in pulmonary hypertension
- Use of CPET for diagnosis and clinical follow-up

CLASSIFICATION OF ETIOLOGIES OF PULMONARY HYPERTENSION

Pulmonary hypertension (PH) is defined by increased pressures (resting mean PAP > 25 mmHg)

across the pulmonary vasculature, due to either pulmonary vascular disease or elevated left atrial pressures. Patients with pulmonary hypertension have been divided into five diagnostic groups:

Group 1: Pulmonary artery hypertension including idiopathic, heritable, scleroderma, and drug-associated causes
Group 2: Pulmonary hypertension due to any cause of chronic elevation of left atrial pressure
Group 3: Pulmonary arterial hypertension due to underlying lung disease such as COPD or interstitial lung disease
Group 4: Pulmonary arterial hypertension secondary to chronic thromboembolic disease
Group 5: Pulmonary arterial hypertension due to miscellaneous hematologic causes

While there are some common elements of exercise responses among all of these pulmonary hypertension groups, this chapter focuses on the exercise responses of Group 1 and Group 4 patients.

CLINICAL PRESENTATION OF PATIENTS WITH PAH

The classic presentation for a patient with Group 1 PAH is a progressive increase in exertional dyspnea over time, with an associated loss of overall exercise tolerance and generalized fatigue. With progression, patients may note chest pain and exertional lightheadedness. The latter symptom may advance to frank exertional syncope, an ominous symptom suggestive of advanced disease. As the response to drug treatment is better in early-stage disease, the diagnostic use of CPET to identify disease in patients with unexplained dyspnea can lead to an earlier correct diagnosis. Unfortunately, many patients are not identified for over two years, by which time the pulmonary vascular pathology has progressed to a point in which drug treatment is less effective.

PATTERN OF CPET RESPONSE FOR PULMONARY HYPERTENSION PATIENTS

Symptomatic pulmonary hypertension patients undergoing a diagnostic CPET demonstrate a typical pattern of cardiac, ventilation, and gas exchange responses. For patients with severe disease and exertional syncope, a maximal exercise test is obviously contraindicated, but for patients undergoing a diagnostic workup for exertional dyspnea in which pulmonary hypertension is a potential diagnosis, recall that the usual exercise testing precautions for blood pressure and patient monitoring during the test are particularly important.

As with patients with left heart failure, patients with right ventricular impairment from pulmonary hypertension show a reduction in maximal oxygen uptake that is proportional to their disease severity. As with left heart failure patients, they exhibit a ventilatory threshold that can be identified between 60% and 80% of a maximal effort. A striking feature of the cardiac exercise response for a pulmonary hypertension patient is the high resting heart rate and, throughout the exercise test, an associated low O_2 pulse. For patients with severe pulmonary hypertension, the O_2 pulse during exercise may fail to increase despite increasing oxygen consumption, a feature suggesting a progressive loss of right ventricular stroke volume with exercise effort.

A characteristic feature of the exercise response of a pulmonary hypertension patient is both high resting ventilation and an exceptionally brisk ventilation response to exercise. The example below compares the exercise ventilation of a pulmonary hypertension patient with a size- and age-matched subject, illustrating both the lower maximal exercise capacity and the high ventilation response to exercise (Figure 9.1).

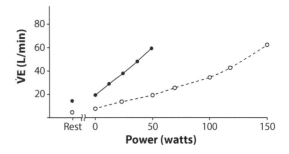

Figure 9.1 High exercise ventilation both at rest and with exercise in a pulmonary hypertension patient (solid dots) compared with a normal subject (open dots).

The high ventilation response arises for two reasons. First, the diffuse pulmonary vascular damage produces small regions within the lung that are poorly perfused but still well ventilated, increasing the physiologic dead space within the lung. Second, the high pulmonary artery pressures and/or the associated right ventricular failure increase the ventilatory drive both at rest and during exercise, and the exercise test measurements of both end-tidal CO_2 and arterial CO_2 are consistently low throughout the test. The $\dot{V}E/\dot{V}CO_2$ ratio, the ventilatory equivalent for CO_2, remains high throughout the exercise response, usually above 35 liters/liter, and sometimes over 50 liters/liter. Despite the high levels of ventilation produced at a given level of oxygen consumption or carbon dioxide output, these patients do not approach a true mechanical limitation of ventilatory capacity, but only because their limitation of cardiac output is proportionately more severe.

EXERCISE GAS EXCHANGE IN PULMONARY HYPERTENSION

While arterial blood gas measurements are not always included with many CPET studies, they are important to obtain in any diagnostic setting when pulmonary hypertension is among the diagnoses under consideration. While patients with pulmonary hypertension generally show a compensated respiratory alkalosis with $PaCO_2$ values in the low 30 mmHg range at rest and with exercise, the most characteristic change is the failure to develop the normal decrease in physiologic dead space during exercise.

Calculation of physiologic dead space

Correct calculation of the physiologic dead space (V_D/V_T) requires the measured $PaCO_2$ and the mean expired CO_2 (P_ECO_2). (Recall that P_ECO_2 is different from the exercise system-presented end-tidal CO_2 [$P_{ET}CO_2$].)

$$V_D/V_T = (PaCO_2 - P_ECO_2)/PaCO_2$$

The P_ECO_2 is calculated from the measurements of $\dot{V}CO_2$ and $\dot{V}E$ at the exercise stage when the blood gases are drawn.

$$P_ECO_2 = k* \dot{V}CO_2/\dot{V}E, \text{ where } k = 863 \text{ mmHg}$$

The "k" converts the fractional concentration of CO_2 in the exhaled breath to mm Hg and corrects for the temperature differences for the calculated $\dot{V}CO_2$ (T = 273°C) and the calculated $\dot{V}E$ (T = 310°C). Some CPET computer systems include a subroutine that will make this V_D/V_T calculation if the measured $PaCO_2$ values are entered into the system (Figure 9.2).

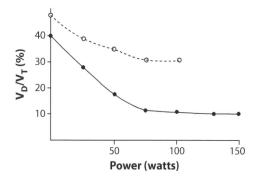

Figure 9.2 Changes in physiologic dead space during exercise in a pulmonary hypertension patient (open circles) and a normal subject (dots).

Figure 9.2 compares the physiologic dead space measurement during exercise made in a pulmonary hypertension patient compared with a subject of the same size and age. Note that, while the physiologic dead space progressively decreases for the normal subject during exercise because their anatomic dead space becomes a smaller and smaller fraction of each breath as exercise progresses, the pulmonary hypertension patient starts with higher dead space and fails to decrease the physiologic dead space during exercise, despite normal increases in tidal volume. This characteristic exercise abnormality is due to the elevated alveolar dead space from pulmonary vascular damage and the very high ventilation relative to the restricted cardiac output.

A second gas exchange abnormality seen in pulmonary hypertension patients during exercise is an increased alveolar-arterial oxygen difference, (A-a)DO_2. Although the arterial PaO_2 may remain in a near-normal range with exercise despite the presence on increased ventilation-perfusion mismatch, it is associated with a low $PaCO_2$, leading to an abnormal (A-a)DO_2 (Figure 9.3). In addition, some pulmonary hypertension patients may develop a right-to-left shunt during exercise from a patent foramen ovale and, in that setting, will demonstrate much more dramatic oxygen desaturation as exercise progresses.

Calculation of the alveolar-arterial O_2 difference

Calculation of the alveolar-arterial O_2 difference ([A-a]DO_2) requires the measured PaO_2 and $PaCO_2$, the respiratory "R" value ($\dot{V}CO_2/\dot{V}O_2$) measured at the time when the blood gases were drawn, and the inspired partial pressure of oxygen (PIO_2). The PIO_2 at sea level (with PB of 760 mmHg), corrected for water vapor pressure, is 150 mmHg.

$$PAO_2 = PIO_2 - PaCO_2/R$$
$$(A-a)DO_2 = PAO_2 - PaO_2$$

A final gas exchange abnormality seen in pulmonary hypertension patients during exercise is related to the difference between a measured $PaCO_2$ and the exercise system-reported end-tidal PCO_2 ($P_{ET}CO_2$). In normal subjects, the $P_{ET}CO_2$ is quite close to the $PaCO_2$ at rest, but with maximal exercise, the $P_{ET}CO_2$ may be as much as 6 mmHg higher than the $PaCO_2$. In pulmonary hypertension, because of the high V_A/Q regions from vascular damage, the $P_{ET}CO_2$ remains lower than the $PaCO_2$ for these patients throughout exercise.

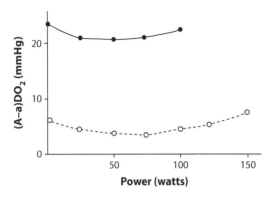

Figure 9.3 Changes in (A-a)DO$_2$ during exercise in a pulmonary hypertension patient (solid dots) and a normal subject (open circles).

Although the above examples show arterial blood gas samples acquired throughout an exercise study, the gas exchange abnormalities most characteristic of pulmonary hypertension are seen at maximal effort, and a simpler approach is to do an arterial puncture immediately after the maximal effort in lieu of placing an arterial catheter for multiple samples throughout the test. (Of course, that assumes the arterial puncture will be successful immediately after the test.)

USE OF CPET FOR DIAGNOSIS AND CLINICAL FOLLOW-UP

While pulmonary hypertension does represent heart failure of the right ventricle and, in common with ordinary cardiac failure, demonstrates a reduced maximal oxygen uptake and a reduced ventilatory threshold, the gas exchange abnormalities are different. Patients with compensated heart failure do not demonstrate an abnormal (A-a)DO$_2$ with exercise. While patients with severe heart failure do demonstrate an elevated $\dot{V}E/\dot{V}CO_2$, the $\dot{V}E/\dot{V}CO_2$ in pulmonary hypertension patients becomes elevated far earlier in their clinical course and reaches levels with severe disease seldom seen with primary left heart failure.

For patients with proven pulmonary hypertension undergoing drug treatment, the only commonly used exercise test is the 6-minute walk. The latter test is convenient for office use and is most effective for the most severely impaired patients. However for workup of patients with relatively mild impairment, the 6-minute walk distance provides no diagnostic information and is poorly correlated with the maximal oxygen uptake of moderately impaired patients. We believe that a standard CPET with arterial blood gas measurement provides a better clinical baseline for initial evaluation of those patients. For patients who have not responded to drug treatment and may be considered for heart-lung transplant, the CPET measurement of O$_2$ pulse with submaximal exercise provides prognostic information. An abnormal O$_2$ pulse response to submaximal exercise identifies a patient group with very high mortality.

SUMMARY POINTS

Exercise testing is an essential component of the investigation of a patient with new exertional dyspnea who may have early pulmonary hypertension. Although the pattern of routine CPET response is helpful in advancing the diagnosis, the acquisition of exercise arterial blood gases significantly improves that diagnostic sensitivity for PAH. As described in this chapter, the most useful findings include

- Severe exertional dyspnea as a subjective symptom

- Decreased aerobic capacity
- Early tachycardia
- Low O$_2$ pulse ($\dot{V}O_2$/heart rate)
- Elevated $\dot{V}E/\dot{V}CO_2$ at rest, exercise, and recovery
- Elevated and abnormal pattern of V$_D$/V$_T$ during exercise
- Exercise hypoxemia or increased A-aDO$_2$

A note: The pattern of exercise limitation described above in early PAH is nearly identical to the pattern observed in early interstitial lung disease, and for that reason, the above exercise abnormalities are described as a combined PAH/ILD pattern requiring additional medical workup for differentiation. Hence for patients exhibiting this constellation of exercise findings, an echocardiogram and right-heart catheterization are essential parts of the subsequent workup. For PAH patients, early diagnosis improves the likely response to treatment and ultimate prognosis.

10

Exercise testing patients with airflow obstruction

Disorders causing airflow obstruction constitute a common cause of exercise limitation, and the pathophysiology of that exercise impairment revealed during a CPET will be discussed here. While COPD and asthma are the most common obstructive diagnoses, laryngeal abnormalities or upper airway abnormalities can also limit exercise performance. Hence the initial clinical evaluation of the patient, which includes appropriate history, physical exam, imaging, and pulmonary function tests, is an important prelude to the exercise study. Although in some cases the cause of dyspnea or exercise limitation is obviously attributable to a severe obstructive abnormality, in patients with mild or moderate airflow obstruction, there are exercise test findings that may suggest a contribution to the overall symptomatic limitation.

- Chronic obstructive pulmonary disease (COPD)
- Exercise-induced bronchospasm
- Laryngeal and upper airway abnormalities

COPD

The range of functional impairment from COPD covers a wide spectrum, ranging from nearly asymptomatic individuals to homebound patients dependent on supplemental oxygen to accomplish the most basic tasks of self-care. Ordinarily, the appropriate pulmonary function testing for a new COPD patient is limited to spirometry, oximetry, and a walk test; however, when the degree of functional impairment seems greater than would

be suggested from the standard clinical evaluation, full exercise testing will provide additional information.

Exercise test findings in COPD

- CPET findings in severe COPD-ventilation limitation
- Dynamic hyperinflation
- Gas exchange
- Peripheral muscle dysfunction
- Cardiopulmonary interaction
- Dyspnea
- Results of a CPET and their use

CPET findings in severe COPD-ventilation limitation

The defining abnormality of COPD is a reduction in maximal expiratory flow rates, quantitated by reduction in the maximal volume of air that can be exhaled in one second, the FEV_1. The effect of this flow reduction on exercise ventilation capacity is best illustrated by a comparison of resting normal and COPD inspiratory and expiratory flow-volume loops (Figure 10.1).

The COPD inspiratory loop (lower loop, running from residual volume [RV] to total lung capacity [TLC]) is not different from the normal patient loop because the negative pleural pressure generated by a sudden inspiratory effort tethers open the diseased COPD airways. However the expiratory part of the COPD loop (upper loop, running from TLC to RV) becomes different from normal almost immediately after the initiation of

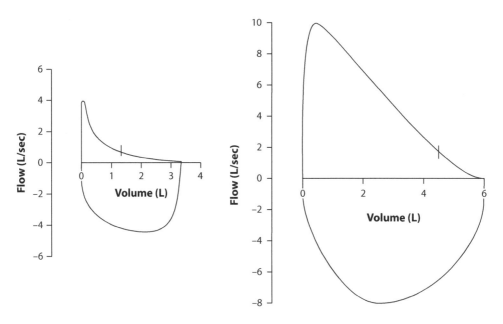

Figure 10.1 Flow-volume loops of a patient with severe COPD (left plot) and a normal subject of the same age and height (right plot). The vertical bar on each expiratory loop marks the portion of the vital capacity exhaled in the first second.

forced exhalation, as the diseased airways narrow rapidly as pleural pressure becomes more positive. Note that, for the patient with COPD, a smaller fraction of the total vital capacity breath is exhaled during the first second of exhalation (the FEV_1) in comparison with the normal subject. The low expiratory flow rate for the COPD patient cannot be improved with more effort, posing a limit to the maximal exercise ventilation. For patients with severe COPD (FEV_1 less than 50% predicted), maximal exercise is impaired by the inability

of ventilation to keep pace with the increasing exercise CO_2 production, leading to progressive increases in arterial and end-tidal CO_2 at maximal effort. In essence, severe COPD patients experience an episode of acute respiratory failure with acute respiratory acidosis during any sustained maximal exercise effort. However, unlike a COPD exacerbation, the respiratory acidosis these patients experience with exertion is due to a two- to four-fold increase in CO_2 production and is readily resolved by stopping the exercise activity (Figure 10.2).

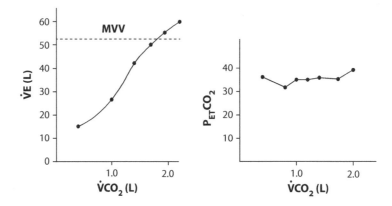

Figure 10.2 CPET ventilation data from a patient with severe COPD showing progression of minute ventilation compared with previously measured MVV (left plot) and progression of end-tidal PCO_2 measurements (right plot).

The minute ventilation that a severe COPD patient achieves with a maximal exercise effort is compared with the resting measurements made of the maximal voluntary ventilation (MVV) and also the estimated MVV obtained by multiplying FEV_1 by 35. (For COPD patients, $FEV_1 \times 35$ represents a better estimate of MVV compared with the $FEV_1 \times 40$ estimate used for subjects without airflow obstruction.) Unlike normal subjects, there is no ventilatory reserve available for maximal exercise, and if a patient reaches their MVV and/or the $FEV_1 \times 35$ during an exercise test, it provides one criterion for a primary ventilation limitation to maximal exercise. (Recall that maximally exercising normal subjects have exercise ventilation that only reaches about 60%–70% of their previously measured MVV.) The resting measurements of MVV and the $FEV_1 \times 35$ are not perfect markers of maximal exercise ventilation. Particularly for patients with very severe airflow obstruction, some patients will consistently exceed those criteria in multiple tests, and some will consistently fail to reach those markers despite an apparent maximal effort.

A second criterion for ventilatory limitation during exercise is the inability to initiate a compensatory respiratory alkalosis (as manifested by a decreasing end-tidal CO_2) during a maximal sustained effort. Although the end-tidal measurements of CO_2 during exercise for COPD patients are not accurate representations of their arterial CO_2 values, a decreasing end-tidal CO_2 ($ETCO_2$) at maximal effort does reflect end-exercise decreases in arterial PCO_2. Hence, the failure of a COPD patient to decrease $ETCO_2$ at maximal effort, or even increase $ETCO_2$ with maximal effort, represents an unequivocal sign of a primary respiratory limitation to maximal exercise (Figure 10.2).

An exercise ventilation pattern characteristic of all COPD patients is a relatively smaller exercise tidal volume relative to their forced vital capacity. During heavy exercise, normal subjects will have tidal volumes that reach about 60%–70% of their measured forced vital capacity, whereas COPD patients will use a smaller fraction of their FVC. The exercise tidal volumes in COPD patients may actually decrease at the highest tolerated level of exercise (Figure 10.3).

Dynamic hyperinflation

While multiple mechanisms contribute to the overall exercise impairment experienced by patients

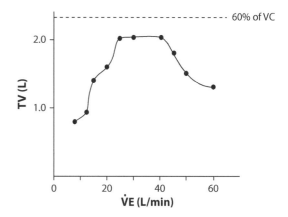

Figure 10.3 Progression of tidal volume in a severe COPD patient during exercise. Dashed line marks 60% of the measured vital capacity.

with COPD, exercise-associated air trapping or dynamic hyperinflation is the most important. COPD is defined by the reduction in expiratory flow rates, and this impairment becomes the limiting factor for the increased ventilation requirements of exercise. As illustrated below, where a patient's exercise flow volume loop has been superimposed on their pre-exercise maximal flow volume loop, the exercise tidal volume loop impinges on the maximal expiratory loop throughout exhalation. As flow cannot be increased at lower lung volumes, the only option for increasing expiratory flow is to make a bigger inspiratory effort, so that each exhalation begins at a higher lung volume (Figure 10.4).

With the exercise-associated increase in respiratory rate, the available time for exhalation decreases, and the only way a COPD patient can increase expiratory flow rates during exercise is to inspire to a higher lung volume, and in turn that requirement increases the work of breathing. This inability to completely exhale back to the resting FRC as the respiratory rate increases is termed dynamic hyperinflation (DH). During a progressive exercise test, measurements of inspiratory capacity (IC) can reveal the existence of DH. During the exercise effort, the patient is periodically asked to make a maximal inspiratory effort at the beginning of a normal exercise breath and resume normal breathing. The volume of that breath will be the exercise IC. For normal subjects performing heavy exercise, their IC will increase from the resting measurement, as they then begin their exercise breaths below their resting FRC. For most subjects with even mild to moderate COPD,

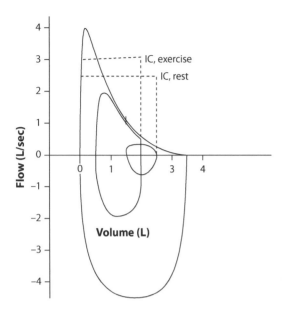

Figure 10.4 Maximal flow-volume loop in a severe COPD patient measured at rest, with superimposed resting tidal volume loop (smallest loop) and an exercise tidal volume loop (middle loop). The dotted lines mark the inspiratory capacity (IC) measured at rest and the IC measured at maximal exercise.

the exercise inspiratory capacity will become smaller than their resting IC because of dynamic hyperinflation. For subjects with more severe COPD, dynamic hyperinflation is a uniform finding, but with some variability in severity among individuals that may explain the differences in exercise capacity among COPD patients who have similarly impaired values of FEV_1.

Dynamic hyperinflation substantially increases the work of breathing because breathing during

heavy exercise requires inspiration to a high fraction of the total lung capacity. Continuously inspiring to a high a lung volume both increases the work of breathing and puts a heavier load on the accessory muscles of ventilation, as the flattened diaphragms of COPD patients at high lung volumes lose some of their mechanical advantage. Studies have described severe subjective dyspnea for COPD patients during exercise when their exercise tidal volume approaches 75% of their exercise IC. Exercise studies of COPD patients with lesser degrees of airflow obstruction may not show classic signs of ventilatory limitation based on the criteria of reaching their MVV or failing to decrease their end-tidal CO_2 with maximal effort, but still show decreasing exercise inspiratory capacity. These patients frequently describe dyspnea as their limiting subjective symptom. Although documenting a reproducible decrease in inspiratory capacity may be difficult for an exercising COPD patient, the secondary finding that maximal exercise tidal volumes are consistently smaller than the normal 50%–60% of the resting vital capacity is at least suggestive of dynamic hyperinflation.

Gas exchange

The hallmark of COPD is impaired exchange of both oxygen and carbon dioxide. These abnormalities arise because of the mismatch between blood flow and ventilation throughout the COPD lung, whereby low VA/Q regions produce hypoxemia and high VA/Q regions impair the efficiency of carbon dioxide elimination (Figure 10.5).

Figure 10.5 shows a distribution of lung regions sorted by VA/Q ratio for a normal lung and a COPD

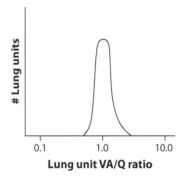
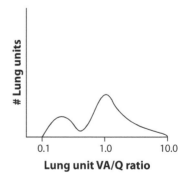

Figure 10.5 The distribution of VA/Q ratios within multiple same-sized volumes of a normal lung (left plot) and the distribution of VA/Q ratios within a COPD lung. Note the COPD lung has units with a low VA/Q ratios (producing hypoxemia) and high ratios (contributing to physiologic dead space).

lung. The lowest VA/Q units in the normal lung still have capillary O_2 saturations of greater than 90%, whereas the low VA/Q units in the COPD lung have saturations in the 70%–75% range, very close to the saturation in mixed venous blood when a patient is at rest. For the COPD lung, the contribution from low VA/Q units brings the overall arterial saturation down to the 85%–90% range. With exercise, the normal progressive reduction of mixed venous oxygen saturation further reduces the oxygen saturation in the low VA/Q units and may further decrease the overall arterial saturation. While the (A-a) O_2 difference is increased in nearly all COPD patients, there is substantial variability among patients in the severity of their hypoxemia at rest and with exercise. Some of this individual variability appears to be related to inborn respiratory drives, as patients with blunted ventilation drives tend to show the most marked hypoxemia, whereas some COPD patients with very brisk ventilation drives may show only mild hypoxemia with exercise but experience severe dyspnea.

The carbon dioxide gas exchange abnormalities in patients with mild or moderate COPD are hidden, as they have normal values for arterial PCO_2, although they require abnormally high exercise ventilation to maintain that normal $PaCO_2$. This loss of ventilation efficiency is a consequence of the broad VA/Q distribution for COPD patients illustrated above, whereas the abnormality in CO_2 exchange is primarily attributable to the high VA/Q units. (The high VA/Q units have very low alveolar CO_2 partial pressures that dilute the overall alveolar PCO_2, producing an effect indistinguishable from the influence of the anatomic dead space on overall gas exchange.) For COPD patients, the exercise physiologic dead space is increased because of the disproportionate contribution of high VA/Q units to the total ventilation. Hence, for mild or moderate COPD patients who can maintain normal or near-normal arterial PCO_2 values during exercise, the high physiologic dead space gives them both a high resting $\dot{V}E/\dot{V}CO_2$ and abnormally high $\dot{V}E/\dot{V}CO_2$ values in the range of 35–50 liters/liter throughout the exercise performance. However, for COPD patients with more severe obstruction, whose exercise ventilation cannot keep pace with their CO_2 production, their early exercise high $\dot{V}E/\dot{V}CO_2$ values decrease progressively as they approach their absolute ventilatory limit, associated with a stable or increasing end-tidal CO_2 (Figure 10.6).

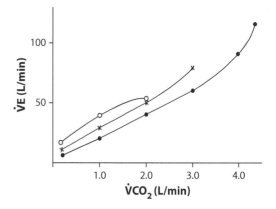

Figure 10.6 $\dot{V}E/\dot{V}CO_2$ exercise plots for a normal subject (solid dots), a moderate COPD patient ("x") and a severe COPD patient (open circles). Note only the normal subject shows end-exercise augmentation of ventilation, and that the severe COPD patient begins with the steepest slope that then flattens out.

Peripheral muscle function

Patients with mild COPD will frequently describe leg fatigue rather than dyspnea as their primary limiting symptom, and as a group, mild COPD patients will have lower maximal oxygen uptakes than comparable subjects without COPD. Although patients with more severe COPD have an almost universal complaint of dyspnea as their limiting symptom, they also show signs of peripheral muscle abnormalities characterized by many of the features of deconditioning and disuse atrophy: diminished muscle mass, reduced aerobic oxidative capacity, and decreased mitochondrial and capillary density. While the severe COPD patients are so limited that severe muscle deconditioning would be expected, it is plausible that there is some skeletal muscle abnormality associated with all COPD beyond simple deconditioning that provides a secondary limit to their maximal exercise performance. However, even the most severely affected patients can improve some of these muscle abnormalities with training. Improved sustained work capacity, moving the lactate threshold to a higher level of work, and increasing capillary and mitochondrial density in working muscles have all been documented to occur with patient training and are the same types of improvement any normal individual will undergo with sustained training.

Cardiopulmonary interactions in COPD

For patients with severe COPD, associated cardiac impairment also limits overall exercise tolerance. Apart from the obvious coronary artery disease risks from cigarette smoking, the right heart has limitations imposed by severe COPD. Untreated chronic hypoxia leads to pulmonary hypertension and right heart failure, but even for patients treated with supplemental oxygen, increased pulmonary vascular resistance remains a problem that is more apparent during exercise. For patients with significant pulmonary hypertension, the additional stimulus of exercise will increase right ventricular volume and impinge on the interventricular septum, impairing left ventricular stroke volume. In addition, the development of dynamic hyperinflation during exercise will produce intermittent positive intrathoracic pressure, impairing venous return. Although multifactorial, any combination of these abnormalities leads to further impairment of cardiac output, manifested by a low O_2 pulse that fails to increase appropriately with progressive exercise.

Dyspnea

As shortness of breath is a primary limiting symptom in exercise, it can be quantitated and also followed as patients undertake training with rehabilitation or treatment with bronchodilators or oxygen. Analog scales to document the severity of the subjective sense of dyspnea are useful tools to follow patients undergoing pulmonary rehabilitation to document objective improvement and provide psychological encouragement.

Use of CPET in COPD

While FEV_1 measurements are used to document the relative severity of COPD and choose treatment options, it is nevertheless true that for any given level of airflow obstruction, there are substantial differences in maximal exercise capacity. For patients with disproportionate exercise impairment, a CPET may reveal unexpected dynamic hyperinflation, exercise-associated hypoxemia, or a primary unanticipated cardiac impairment. Understanding the components of the exercise response can help the practitioner focus on the important aspects of

the patient's pathophysiology and consider therapeutic interventions based on that information. For instance, exercise flow-volume loops or inspiratory capacity measurements acquired during progressive or steady-state exercise provide documentation of dynamic hyperinflation, where even small improvements in airflow from bronchodilators are beneficial to reduce the degree of dynamic hyperinflation. For patients demonstrating exercise desaturation, oxygen therapy has beneficial effects on performance by reducing respiratory rate and thereby diminishing the severity of dynamic hyperinflation. The information gained from exercise testing helps to select the therapeutic modalities packaged in a comprehensive COPD rehabilitation program that can result in a more satisfactory quality of life for patients whose disease can limit performance of even the simplest activities of daily living.

EXERCISE-INDUCED BRONCHOSPASM (EIB)

Many patients with a clinical diagnosis of asthma are aware that their asthma symptoms are exacerbated by exercise. However exacerbation of asthma symptoms with heavy exercise is not a universal symptom of all patients with reversible airflow obstruction. On the other hand, many individuals without a clinical history suggestive of asthma may present with new dyspnea, associated with wheezing and cough, that is triggered by exercise. These subjects are commonly healthy, active physically, and nonsmokers without known allergies. Their resting PFTs may be normal. Many are young adolescent or teenage aerobic athletes, although the exercise-related symptoms may begin at any age. While a clinical evaluation is important to rule out other causes, exercise-induced bronchospasm (EIB) is a relatively common diagnosis in this clinical setting.

The increase in sympathetic tone from exercise normally results in a modest degree of bronchodilation in most subjects, so that small increases in FVC and FEV_1 are ordinarily noted a few minutes after a maximal exercise test. However, patients with EIB will demonstrate a progressive decline in FEV_1 during or within 5–30 minutes after heavy exercise, and this abnormality can be reversed by administration of an inhaled bronchodilator. The mechanism triggering EIB in susceptible individuals is any stimulus that dries out the conducting airways. Hence the best stimulus to induce EIB involves performing sustained heavy exercise while breathing perfectly dry air from a hospital air-line or from a compressed air tank. While post-exercise spirometry measurements may reveal EIB after a standard CPET protocol, a more sensitive method to trigger EIB involves a sustained heavy exercise effort: running the patient on a treadmill while breathing dry air, at a fixed speed and grade for the highest level the patient can sustain for 5–6 minutes.

Confirming a suspected diagnosis of diagnosis of EIB is important, as its treatment is ordinarily simple and totally effective in reversing symptoms and returning athletes to peak performance. Beta agonist inhalers used alone before exercise are normally all that is needed; although some individuals may require additional therapy with inhaled cholinergics or oral leukotriene inhibitors.

Several protocols have been suggested to document EIB, all of which involve breathing dry air during heavy ventilation. All involve initial resting spirometry with flow-volume loops (FVL). In addition to the treadmill exercise protocol described above or a maximum CPET, a resting hyperventilation test has been described that requires addition of CO_2 to the inspired air to prevent severe hypocapnea during a period of sustained hyperventilation. Either the exercise or resting hyperventilation challenge is followed by sequential spirometry performed at five, ten, fifteen, and thirty minutes after the end of the EIB challenge. Any decrease in the FEV1 is abnormal and suggestive of EIB, but a 15% decrease in airflow at any point of the test is considered diagnostic of EIB. If a decrease in airflow is present, bronchodilators should then be administered to confirm efficacy of therapy.

VARIABLE UPPER AIRWAY DYSFUNCTION

Some patients with dyspnea on exertion are empirically diagnosed with EIB without a diagnostic workup and are treated unsuccessfully with inhaled

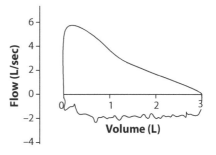

Figure 10.7 Abnormal exercise inspiratory flow loop showing very limited inspiratory flows in a patient with upper airways dysfunction.

bronchodilators. These individuals are often young active athletes, more commonly women than men. Following performance of an EIB challenge that failed to produce airflow obstruction, the differential diagnosis should include variable upper airway dysfunction (VUAD). Documentation of this disorder requires laryngeal endoscopy during exercise, using a flexible nasal endoscope. (It is not diagnostically adequate to perform the endoscopy immediately after exercise because the findings can resolve almost immediately after exercise.) The obstructive abnormality can involve either the supraglottic structures of the larynx or the vocal cords themselves. This disorder has a number of potential etiologies, including psychological conversion reactions, vocal cord irritation from GERD, and post-nasal drip (PND), allergies, or inhalation of environmental irritants.

Flow/volume loops during a CPET may provide a helpful tool initiate a diagnostic workup for VUAD if the inspiratory loop is shallow and flattened during heavy exercise (Figure 10.7).

During the test, sounds of inspiratory stridor may also be diagnostically helpful. VUAD is important to diagnose, although it may be variable in its presentation. It is treatable with appropriate interventions to stop the irritants if it is GERD or other inhaled toxic substances, or speech therapy if no irritant stimulus is apparent.

SUMMARY POINTS

- Patients with severe COPD are limited by their maximal ventilation capacity, where maximal exercise ventilation reaches the previously measured maximal voluntary ventilation or their $FEV_1 \times 35$. At maximal effort, they cannot increase ventilation to produce the normal end-exercise reduction in end-tidal CO_2.

- Patients with less severe COPD may also develop dynamic hyperinflation during exercise, increasing the work of breathing and symptomatic dyspnea, even though they do not demonstrate the classic signs of ventilation limitation.
- Not all patients with asthma will demonstrate exercise-induced bronchospasm (EIB), and some patients will develop only exercise-induced bronchospasm without the other ordinary manifestations of asthma.

EIB is best diagnosed by utilizing a protocol of sustained heavy treadmill exercise while breathing dry air, followed by a timed sequence of post-exercise spirometry measurements.

- While the measurement of flow/volume loops during exercise can provide evidence suggestive of variable upper airways dysfunction, that diagnosis is best established utilizing exercise fiberoptic nasal laryngoscopy.

11

Exercise testing patients with restrictive lung abnormalities

The exercise manifestations seen within the diverse assortment of pulmonary diseases that have a reduced total lung capacity fall into two different patterns of response. The first group includes disorders that produce diffuse pulmonary parenchymal scarring, diseases in which the earliest manifestations may be revealed with a properly conducted CPET. The second group of restrictive disorders arise secondary to respiratory muscle weakness or chest wall abnormalities, but with normal pulmonary parenchyma.

EXERCISE RESPONSES OF PATIENTS WITH INTERSTITIAL LUNG DISEASE

The term interstitial lung disease (ILD) encompasses many different pathological processes, including sarcoidosis, idiopathic pulmonary fibrosis, scleroderma and other connective tissue diseases, hypersensitivity pneumonitis, silicosis, asbestosis, and other lung-scarring disorders. The initial clinical symptom for most of these disorders is increased exertional dyspnea, and it is in the setting of disease onset where a CPET may provide the most useful information. Static pulmonary function tests for all of these disorders eventually show a reduced total lung capacity with a normal FEV_1/FVC ratio and a reduced diffusing capacity. Patients with early ILD may still have normal static pulmonary function measurements, with abnormalities only apparent from data acquired with a CPET.

CPET characteristics of a patient with early ILD

ILD patients with normal or low-normal total lung capacities still may present with symptoms of exertional dyspnea and reduced exercise tolerance, and in this setting, a CPET is most diagnostically useful. The earliest and most characteristic exercise abnormality seen in an ILD patient is an increased exercise ventilatory demand, as demonstrated by an increased exercise $\dot{V}E/\dot{V}CO_2$. However, there is a broad range of normal values for exercise $\dot{V}E/\dot{V}CO_2$, so that obtaining a high-normal value on a patient with new exertional dyspnea is not diagnostically useful unless a lower exercise $\dot{V}E/\dot{V}CO_2$ had been measured previously. Other suggestive early findings include a consistently reduced $ETCO_2$ and a maximal exercise tidal volume that does not reach 60% of the resting vital capacity. However the same reservations for those modest abnormalities also apply: without prior exercise tests showing that those measurements represent a change, they are not helpful (Figure 11.1).

For a patient with new dyspnea of unknown etiology, a CPET that includes measurement of arterial blood gases adds useful information.

Exercise blood gases for the interpretation of an elevated exercise $\dot{V}E/\dot{V}CO_2$

Two different exercise abnormalities can contribute to the elevated $\dot{V}E/\dot{V}CO_2$ observed in patients

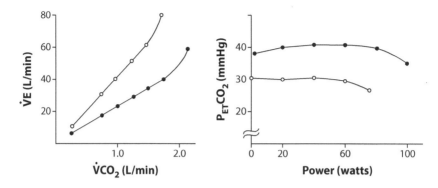

Figure 11.1 $\dot{V}E/\dot{V}CO_2$ and $ETCO_2$ plots of ILD patient and normal patient. $\dot{V}E/\dot{V}CO_2$ and $ETCO_2$ responses of two patients, one with early ILD and one with normal exercise ventilation.

with early ILD. First, ILD patients develop a chronic compensated respiratory alkalosis that persists throughout exercise. This abnormality alone increases the $\dot{V}E/\dot{V}CO_2$, although some normal subjects do have a persistent compensated respiratory alkalosis. However, in ILD, the scarring parenchymal abnormalities create a mismatch between blood flow and ventilation in the lung, and an elevated physiologic dead space measurement is one reflection of that increased VA/Q heterogeneity. Using exercise $PaCO_2$ and exhaled gas CO_2 measurements, the physiologic dead space can be calculated throughout a CPET effort. ILD patients do not show the normal reduction in physiologic V_D/V_T with exercise, and that increased dead space represents the second factor that increases the $\dot{V}E/\dot{V}CO_2$ of ILD patients during exercise (Figure 11.2). For an ILD patient, the low end-tidal PCO_2 seen during an exercise test arises from a combination of hyperventilation and VA/Q mismatch, so the end-tidal PCO_2 measurement does not add new information.

Exercise blood gases and oxygenation in an ILD patient

In early ILD, the arterial O_2 saturation is ordinarily in a normal range during an exercise test. However, while the ventilation-perfusion abnormalities that develop in ILD also impair oxygen uptake in the lung, the abnormality is hidden in early disease because of the chronic hyperventilation. Arterial PO_2 measurements taken during a CPET can be paired with the simultaneous exhaled gas measurement of the respiratory R ($\dot{V}CO_2/\dot{V}O_2$) and the arterial PCO_2 to calculate an alveolar-arterial

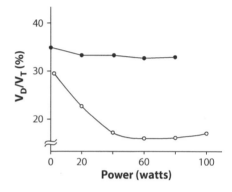

Figure 11.2 V_D/V_T during exercise in a normal subject and an idiopathic pulmonary fibrosis patient.

O_2 difference. In a normal subject, this difference decreases to less than 10 mmHg during exercise, whereas even in early ILD it remains above 20 mmHg (Figure 11.3).

Exercise findings in patients with progressive ILD

With progression of scarring abnormalities from any of the ILD diagnoses, the elevated $\dot{V}E/\dot{V}CO_2$ remains a persistent abnormality, with very substantial increases in the range of 40–60 liters/liter CO_2 that may also be driven further by the exercise-associated hypoxemia that develops with severe disease. Those factors make identifying a ventilatory threshold nearly impossible without sampling arterial blood for lactate levels. With severe disease, some element of pulmonary hypertension develops. Furthermore, in both sarcoidosis and progressive systemic sclerosis, primary myocardial

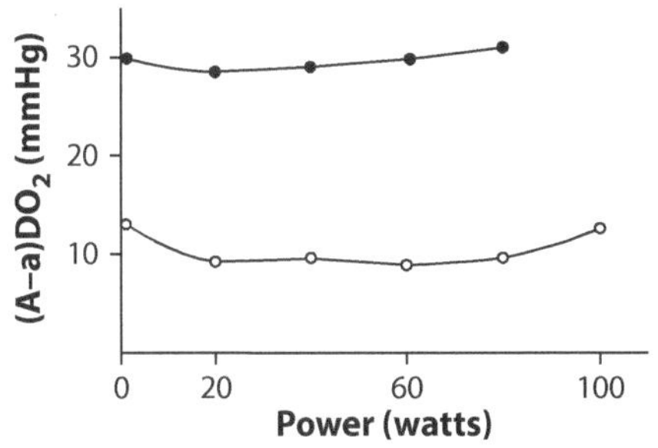

Figure 11.3 (A-a)O_2 difference during exercise in a normal subject (open circles) and an idiopathic pulmonary fibrosis patient (closed circles).

involvement may also be present. Either of those abnormalities will produce a low exercise cardiac output and a low O_2 pulse. The profound exercise limitation seen in patients with advanced ILD disease almost always has some component of pulmonary hypertension and right heart failure. Finally, in severe disease, the combination of the restrictive pulmonary abnormality and the high physiologic dead space may manifest terminally as an elevated arterial $PaCO_2$. In the management of patients with severe ILD, the CPET only offers an index of the severity of the impairment, and this information can be more easily obtained from the much simpler six-minute walk test.

EXERCISE RESPONSES IN PATIENTS WITH RESTRICTIVE VENTILATION IMPAIRMENT WITH NORMAL LUNG PARENCHYMA

The exercise pattern of mechanical ventilatory restriction

The pattern of mechanical restriction to exercise ventilation arises either because of respiratory muscle weakness and/or chest wall abnormalities that increase the work of ventilation. Recall that with a maximal exercise effort, normal subjects will reach minute ventilation somewhere between 60%–80% of their previously measured maximal voluntary ventilation (MVV). (An estimate of the MVV can be obtained by multiplying the FEV_1 by 40.) Using either the MVV or $FEV_1 \times 40$ estimate, the difference between that estimate and exercise ventilation measured at the end of the CPET is termed the ventilatory reserve. Hence, during a maximal exercise effort, a ventilatory reserve of less than 10% of the MVV at least raises suspicion for a mechanical ventilation impairment that could contribute to a patient's overall exercise limitation.

Unilateral or bilateral diaphragm paralysis

While there is a surprising range of maximal exercise capacity among patients with fluoroscopically documented unilateral diaphragmatic paralysis, the overwhelming majority of these patients describe dyspnea as their primary limiting symptom during heavy exercise. When studied with a CPET, they demonstrate the classic signs of exercise ventilation limitation. The maximal exercise ventilation that they attain is very close to both their maximal voluntary ventilation (MVV), so that their ventilatory reserve is nearly zero. In addition, as these patients approach a symptom-limited maximal exercise effort, their exercise end-tidal PCO_2 remains constant or may even increase at maximal effort.

These patients will show a normal or even moderately decreased ventilatory equivalent for CO_2 ($\dot{V}E/\dot{V}CO_2$) during the submaximal exercise portion of their test and ordinarily demonstrate an identifiable ventilatory threshold before attaining their maximal exercise effort. While the majority of diaphragmatic paralysis patients show a very small ventilatory reserve with a maximal effort, a minority can demonstrate a normal cardiovascular limitation pattern, including a reduction in end-tidal CO_2 at maximal effort and at least some ventilatory reserve at end-exercise. Nevertheless, even these less-impaired patients describe severe subjective dyspnea during heavy exercise.

Chest wall abnormalities

Patients with pectus excavatum generally have mild restrictive abnormalities, with vital capacity measurements in the 70%–80% range of predicted value for their height. During CPET testing, they show a modestly reduced maximal oxygen uptake, although the degree of that limitation is variable. While they demonstrate a reduced ventilatory reserve, they also show a significantly reduced O_2 pulse despite a normal maximal exercise heart rate, an indication of a reduced stroke volume. The pectus deformity can create an external restriction to normal cardiac filling, and for many of the patients, this stroke volume limitation is the primary factor determining their reduced maximal oxygen uptake. Paired exercise studies of pectus excavatum children before and after corrective surgery for the abnormality demonstrated a significant postoperative increase in their maximal oxygen uptake, with a lower heart rate at each exercise work load, suggesting an improvement in exercise stroke volume. While the surgery did not significantly improve resting pulmonary function measurements, for any given exercise workload, the children also had higher minute ventilation with less subjective dyspnea compared with their preoperative measurements. This observation suggested that the pectus deformity imposed an increased mechanical load on exercise ventilation in addition to the well-documented pectus-induced limitation in ventricular filling.

Adults with surgically corrected congenital heart disease usually required thoracic surgery interventions in infancy, creating a mild-to-moderate restrictive pulmonary abnormality that persists into adulthood. However, none of those individuals show an exercise limitation suggestive of ventilatory limitation. To some extent, this lack of a ventilatory impairment is attributable to limitations of the cardiac surgical corrections, so that maximal exercise ventilation is lower because of a lower maximal cardiac output. However, even for the adult congenital heart disease patients who have normal maximal oxygen uptakes (as can be seen with some patients with corrected Tetralogy of Fallot), their exercise performance is not limited by restriction of ventilation.

Patients with restrictive abnormalities secondary to kyphoscoliosis have a range of exercise ventilation impairment that correlates with the severity of the scoliosis. Patients with severe curvature abnormalities that approach a 90° bend in the spine represent the most severely limited group. These patients at maximal tolerated exercise demonstrate no ventilatory reserve, and develop a progressive increase in end-tidal CO_2 during a maximal exercise effort.

SUMMARY POINTS

- Exertional dyspnea is the initial symptom of almost all ILD patients, and a CPET is most useful in that early stage of disease. The initial abnormality seen with a CPET is an increased $\dot{V}E/\dot{V}CO_2$. However, at the early stages of disease, exercise arterial blood gases are required to determine whether or not there is an elevated exercise physiologic dead space and an elevated $(A-a)O_2$ difference.
- With progression of any ILD, pulmonary hypertension, exercise-associated hypoxemia, the high $\dot{V}E/\dot{V}CO_2$ and increased work of breathing all contribute to the severe impairment.

- As noted in Chapter 9, the pattern of CPET abnormalities in patients with early ILD cannot be distinguished from the CPET pattern seen in patients with pulmonary hypertension, and an echocardiogram remains in important additional study for a patient whose CPET findings are consistent with early ILD.
- Patients with respiratory muscle or chest wall abnormalities ordinarily describe dyspnea as an exercise-limiting symptom, but depending on the underlying abnormality may demonstrate a wide range of overall exercise impairment.

12

Exercise testing patients with metabolic myopathies

Among the overwhelming variety of rare inherited disorders causing abnormalities of intracellular energy production, a much smaller subset of these patients present in adulthood with the primary symptom of progressive exercise intolerance. These uncommon patients constitute the most likely group of the metabolic myopathies to be referred for diagnostic exercise testing as part of their initial workup. While a CPET will not establish a specific diagnosis, the pattern of exercise limitation may at least raise suspicion for one of these muscle metabolic defects and suggest whether the cellular abnormality is intra- or extra-mitochondrial in nature.

Patients with primary muscle metabolic abnormalities demonstrate reduced maximal oxygen uptake and a relatively low maximal exercise heart rate. For the few metabolic myopathy patients in which the CPET study has included either measurements of exercise cardiac output or measurements including mixed venous saturations from a pulmonary artery catheter, the calculated or measured mixed venous saturation at maximal effort is substantially higher than the normal 25% range for mixed venous oxygen saturation observed in nearly all subjects giving a maximal effort. The suggested interpretation of this observation is that there is still adequate cardiac output and heart rate reserve available, but the exercising muscle is failing because of a problem with muscle fuel utilization. During a routine CPET, two general categories of abnormality are observed with these patients: abnormal cytoplasmic fuel mobilization or abnormal mitochondrial function.

ABNORMAL CYTOPLASMIC FUEL MOBILIZATION

McArdle disease is the best-recognized muscle metabolic abnormality that produces a severe limitation in sustained exercise performance. These patients are characterized by an inability to generate the normal increase in arterial lactate during a sustained maximal muscular effort. The metabolic defect is in an intramuscular enzyme that is required to initiate the mobilization of skeletal muscle glycogen during heavy exercise. Without the muscle glycogen mobilization needed to increase pyruvate generation and ultimately fuel mitochondrial ATP generation during moderate and heavy exercise, these patients have only fatty acids as mitochondrial fuel sources and are accordingly quite limited in their maximal exercise performance, with maximal oxygen uptakes less than 50% of predicted normal values. Despite the absence of lactate and acidosis with heavy exercise, these patients do demonstrate an appropriate ventilatory threshold, suggesting that the norepinephrine washing out from muscles during heavy exercise also acts to trigger the ventilatory threshold. In addition to showing no significant increase in arterial lactate during a standard CPET, these patients also show an atypical heart rate response that has been termed a "second wind" phenomenon. While undergoing a long-duration CPET (using very small exercise increments), McArdle patients will approach a maximal heart rate within the initial five minutes and then demonstrate a reduction in exercise heart rate as the load progresses until they once again reach a maximal heart rate at 15–20 minutes of exercise.

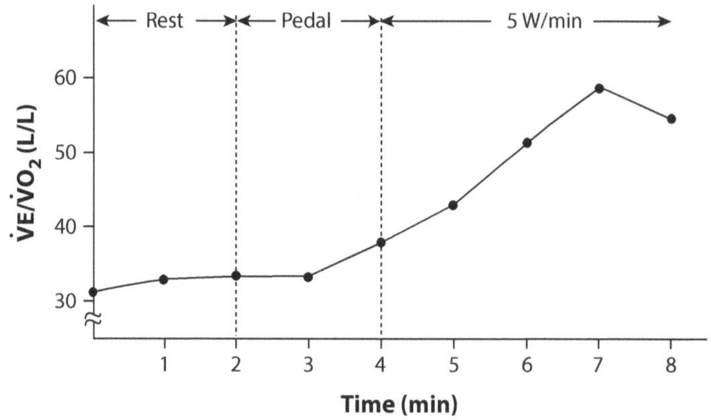

Figure 12.1 Measurements of $\dot{V}E/\dot{V}O_2$ vs. CPET test time for a patient with a mitochondrial myopathy. Note that ventilatory threshold begins during unloaded pedaling and that maximal tolerated exercise using 5-watt increments was 20 watts.

This recovery of exercise capacity during sustained exercise has been attributed to slower onset glycogen mobilization from the liver (instead of exercising muscle) providing a systemic source of glucose for the exercising muscle.

ABNORMAL MITOCHONDRIAL FUNCTION

The many different mitochondrial myopathies in adult patients present a wide range of impairment, from severe limitation to low-normal maximal oxygen uptakes, depending on the mitochondrial defect and duration of the symptomatology. Any of those mitochondrial defects impair the production of the additional ATP needed to support sustained exercise, despite the delivery of adequate oxygen and metabolic fuel to those organelles. Patients with mitochondrial defects will be much more dependent on the anaerobic ATP generation from glycogen mobilization within muscle, and hence during a CPET will demonstrate the very early onset of both lactic acidosis and a ventilatory threshold during their limited CPET capacity (Figure 12.1).

Some muscle mitochondrial myopathy patients will have elevated lactate levels at rest, in addition to the very early onset of arterial lactate during exercise. CPET studies of mitochondrial myopathy patients that include measurements of exercise cardiac output (Q), oxygen consumption ($\dot{V}O_2$), and arterial oxygen content (CaO_2) permit the calculation of mixed venous oxygen content (CvO_2) and mixed venous saturation during maximal exercise.

$$CvO_2 = (\dot{V}O_2/Q) - CaO_2$$

Recall that during a maximal exercise effort, both normal subjects and patients with cardiac disease are able to effectively extract oxygen from the arterial blood, attaining mixed venous O_2 saturations of 25% or less. For the mitochondrial myopathy patients, despite giving a maximal exercise effort, their mixed venous oxygen saturations may remain as high as 50%. This finding suggests that there is more than adequate oxygen delivery to the exercising muscles at maximal effort, but the muscle mitochondria cannot utilize that delivered oxygen for sufficient ATP generation.

SUMMARY POINTS

- Inherited or acquired muscle ATP production abnormalities limit exercise capacity. These uncommon disorders can arise from either abnormalities of fuel mobilization within muscle or abnormalities of mitochondrial function.
- McArdle's syndrome is the commonest fuel mobilization disorder and is

characterized by severe exertional limitation and an inability to mobilize muscle glycogen to support either mitochondrial or anaerobic ATP generation. This abnormality is revealed by an inability to develop lactic acidosis with sustained heavy exercise.

- The muscle mitochondrial abnormalities show exercise limitation with very early lactic acidosis during a CPET, as the mitochondria are unable to adequately increase ATP production with exercise, requiring early utilization of the anaerobic production of ATP from glycolysis.

13

Differential diagnosis for loss of exercise tolerance

Any clinician who performs exercise testing receives a number of referrals for patients who describe an appreciable loss of exercise tolerance developing over a period of weeks or months, without an identified diagnosis. In some cases, the results of the CPET may only reveal a normal cardiovascular pattern of limitation, but with a maximal oxygen uptake that is below what would be expected from the patient's previous exercise baseline. In many of these instances, useful information is gained by repeating the exercise test after a few months when symptoms persist. This chapter presents a list of diagnostic considerations that reflect our combined clinical experience in seeking a diagnosis in this often-challenging clinical scenario.

DIASTOLIC DYSFUNCTION

Documentation of exercise-related diastolic dysfunction is challenging without a pulmonary artery catheter in place. However, a suspicion of this diagnosis is raised by the failure of the O_2 pulse to continue to increase in the final stages of a progressive exercise test. In the case for which a prior resting echocardiogram has shown findings suggestive of diastolic dysfunction and the patient demonstrates that abnormal progression of O_2 pulse during a CPET, the diagnosis of exercise-related diastolic dysfunction is more certain.

SUBCLINICAL HYPOTHYROIDISM

Physically active patients with a mildly elevated TSH and normal-range T4 ordinarily describe a loss of exercise tolerance. The syndrome produces a range of physiologic abnormalities, but most notably in this specific population, it produces a reduction in stroke volume that can be corrected by thyroid supplementation sufficient to drop TSH levels back into a normal range. Many physicians are reluctant to treat this level of deficiency associated with a normal free-T4 measurement, but hormone replacement treatment clearly can yield a measurable improvement in maximal exercise capacity.

OCCULT LOW-LEVEL BLOOD LOSS

While a hemoglobin measurement is ordinarily part of a standard workup for loss of exercise tolerance that is done before requesting a diagnostic CPET, the occasional anemic patient does sneak in. The loss of maximal oxygen uptake from anemia due to chronic low-level blood loss is not strictly proportional to the severity of the anemia. Both stroke volume and circulating plasma volume increase in compensation for a gradual onset of anemia, so that a slow decrease to a 30% reduction in hemoglobin concentration produces less than a 30% drop in maximal oxygen uptake. Nevertheless, correction of that anemia returns the subject to normal function. Thus, a recent hemoglobin measurement is an important part of a CPET evaluation.

IRON DEFICIENCY WITH NORMAL HEMOGLOBIN CONCENTRATION

A normal hemoglobin concentration despite a low ferritin concentration (level below 30 ng/mL) is associated with a relatively early ventilatory threshold and a modest loss in maximal oxygen consumption. This condition of subclinical iron deficiency is quite common for young women because of both normal menstrual blood loss and pregnancies. Very high-mileage runners of either sex may also develop low ferritin from march hemoglobinuria. At least in animal studies of iron deficiency, a treatment response to intravenous iron takes place within 2–3 days, before any significant change in hemoglobin concentration. With iron repletion, humans demonstrate lower serum lactate concentrations at higher workloads and later anaerobic thresholds. These changes occur within two weeks with oral repletion and probably sooner with intravenous iron administration.

OCCULT CORONARY ARTERY DISEASE

While the exercise ECG obtained during a CPET can often make a diagnosis of unsuspected coronary ischemia, normal exercise ECG tracings are not adequately sensitive to exclude the diagnosis. For patients with appropriate risk factors, exercise echocardiography is an appropriate follow-up test.

PRIMARY SINUS NODE FAILURE AND CHRONOTROPIC IMPAIRMENT

Because of the very large range of normal for maximal exercise heart rates, a patient who demonstrates a maximal exercise heart rate more than two standard deviations below a predicted maximal heart rate value still may not represent an abnormality. However, if that maximal exercise heart rate continues to decline with repeat testing over several months, this becomes a far more likely diagnosis, as a normal maximal exercise heart rate decreases less than one beat per year. Sinoatrial exit block may develop during exercise, resulting in a sudden drop to a fixed slower rate.

RECURRENT PULMONARY EMBOLI

Seeding of small volumes of clot from leg veins over weeks to months may produce a stepwise increase in exertional dyspnea without the acute signs and symptoms ordinarily seen in hospitalized patients with large pulmonary emboli. Because of the large range of normal values for exercise $\dot{V}E/\dot{V}CO_2$ during a CPET, a patient with a lesser clot burden may not show a clearly abnormal $\dot{V}E/\dot{V}CO_2$ measurement. For these patients, the best initial tests are an ultrasound examination of their leg veins and a nucleotide ventilation/perfusion lung scan, as the clot burden for these patients may be smaller and a CT pulmonary angiogram may not reveal multiple small clots. However, for patients who show CPET findings suggestive of pulmonary hypertension including an elevated exercise $\dot{V}E/\dot{V}CO_2$ measurement, an echocardiogram will ordinarily reveal some degree of elevated right-sided pressures.

POSTURAL ORTHOSTATIC TACHYCARDIA SYNDROME (POTS)

Advanced cases of POTS will be detected during a CPET by the failure to raise systolic pressure despite a maximal exercise effort. However, as the syndrome develops relatively slowly, the CPET may show only a modest reduction of maximal exercise blood pressure early in the onset of the syndrome that becomes more abnormal with subsequent follow-up testing. Early-stage POTS may be confirmed with tilt table testing and other tests for abnormalities in autonomic vascular function.

ADRENAL INSUFFICIENCY, HYPOTHYROIDISM, HYPERTHYROIDISM, AND PHEOCHROMOCYTOMA

All of these diagnoses cause substantial loss of exercise capacity on a CPET but are ordinarily diagnosed from clinical presentation and exam rather than CPET findings. Nevertheless, with the onset of any of these disorders in a physically active patient, a loss of exercise tolerance may develop before any of the more characteristic clinical signs and laboratory abnormalities become manifest.

EPISODIC LOSS OF EXERCISE TOLERANCE: CARDIAC

If the patient describes intermittent episodes of exercise limitation with an otherwise normal exercise baseline and a maximal oxygen uptake on CPET that fits with that normal baseline, two rhythm-related diagnoses should be considered:

1. Episodic exercise-related atrial fibrillation is seen most frequently in recreational athletes aged 50 and older and may be difficult to document because of its intermittent character. The patients usually describe a sudden loss of speed or power at a level of vigorous activity that they ordinarily can tolerate without limitation. They may not be aware of a fluttering chest sensation.
2. Exercise-related regular supraventricular tachycardia is associated with a similar sudden and generally more dramatic loss of exercise tolerance. These patients are more likely to be aware of a fluttering chest sensation.

EPISODIC LOSS OF EXERCISE TOLERANCE: RESPIRATORY

Dyspnea developing during or after heavy exercise may be related to one of two entities:

1. Exercise-induced bronchospasm (EIB) may be relatively inconsistent, but is more frequently triggered by cold air exposure. A repeat treadmill exercise test protocol specifically designed to reveal EIB is indicated if the routine CPET failed to show suggestive findings.
2. Variable upper airway dysfunction (VUAD) also may be intermittent and is often misdiagnosed as EIB unless a negative test specifically designed to elicit EIB has been performed. Exercise systems that can record exercise flow-volume loops during a CPET may reveal a consistently flat inspiratory loop. A specific diagnosis of VUAD requires fiber-optic visualization of the larynx during exercise.

OVER-TRAINING SYNDROME

This entity is seen in highly competitive aerobic athletes who present with an unexplained decrease in both training and competitive performance and who relentlessly continue intense training without recovery bouts programmed into their routine. CPET testing will reveal a $\dot{V}O_2$ max which may be "normal" but which is well below what would be expected in these high-level athletes. The syndrome is discussed in more detail in Chapter 18, Training.

CHRONIC FATIGUE SYNDROME OR SYSTEMIC EXERTION INTOLERANCE DISEASE

This entity is a clinical diagnosis associated with at least six months of inability to partake in previous physical activities, post-exertional malaise, unrefreshing sleep, some cognitive impairment, but without the autonomic abnormalities that characterize POTS. CPET testing reveals a lower than normal $\dot{V}O_2$ max and a ventilatory threshold that is apparent early in the progressive work test.

MITOCHONDRIAL MYOPATHIES

While the most severe mitochondrial myopathies present in infancy, some lesser mitochondrial abnormalities only become apparent over time during adulthood. They present with a decrease in exercise tolerance and increased dyspnea. A CPET study shows a lower than predicted $\dot{V}O_2$ max and a very early onset of the ventilatory threshold within that reduced exercise performance, suggesting an abnormally early onset of exercise-associated acidosis.

The model generally used to create cardiovascular deconditioning is at least three weeks of bed rest, an intervention that reduces maximal oxygen uptake by about 15% in normal subjects because of a reduction in plasma volume and stroke volume. Larger fractional losses of $\dot{V}O_2$ max are only seen in highly trained athletes undergoing this same deconditioning protocol. The primary requirement for even considering deconditioning as an explanation for loss of exercise tolerance is a history of a sustained and dramatic reduction in ordinary daily activity. For a patient presenting with new exertional limitation, a low $\dot{V}O_2$ max but an otherwise normal-appearing CPET pattern, a diagnosis of "deconditioning" is not appropriate.

14

Gender differences in exercise

The purpose of this chapter is to discuss potential differences in responses to exercise between men and women.

MAXIMAL AEROBIC CAPACITY

Maximal aerobic capacity, expressed in mL O_2/minute, is greater in men than women primarily because of the greater body mass and height in men. This difference between sexes narrows when the $\dot{V}O_2$ is normalized by body weight, and the difference is further minimized when fat-free, lean body mass is used for adjustment of the mL O_2/minute measurement. This latter correction adjusts for the increased fractional proportion of adipose tissue in women. However, even with that correction, men, on average, still have a modestly higher $\dot{V}O_2$ max. The reasons for this persistent, albeit small, difference appear related to the normal lower hemoglobin concentration and oxygen-carrying capacity. Another contributing factor may be a muscle fiber area that is about 85% of muscle fiber area in comparably sized men.

Does this slight decrease in aerobic capacity result in differences in athletic performance? There are certainly other factors, but in some common athletic events, women have slower times. These differences have not decreased a great deal over a number of decades. For instance, competitive running times depending on the event are 6%–15% slower in women; long jump 25% is shorter; road and track cycling are 12% slower, and swimming is 6% slower. The relative advantage of the competitive women swimmers may be related to a buoyancy advantage from a higher percentage of adipose tissue.

In running, another factor has to do with efficiency or running economy. A comparison was made comparing performance-matched men and women marathoners. $\dot{V}O_2$ max was equal at about 60 mL/kg/min, with ventilatory thresholds at about 83% of maximum. The women were also historically better trained, but at comparable submaximum speeds and level of $\dot{V}O_2$, the women had higher heart rates, lactate levels, and respiratory R values (Figure 14.1).

Of note, however, is the decreasing gap in performance between women and men in ultra-endurance events including running, swimming, and cycling. The reasons for this narrowing difference are multi-factorial and not yet thoroughly investigated but may include more efficient fuel utilization and biomechanics in these types of events.

PULMONARY RESPONSE

Women's lungs are about 10% smaller than comparably sized men. The reason for this difference is not clear. Investigators have studied whether or not there is any impairment in gas exchange or lung mechanics in women because of this difference. Women do have a minimal decrease in expiratory flow rates compared with men, but that difference does not influence exercise ventilation responses. Diffusion capacity for carbon monoxide is also slightly lower for height in women, but when values are corrected for their smaller lung size, no difference is appreciated. The most sensitive measurements of exercise gas exchange using the multiple inert gas elimination technique have demonstrated that exercise gas exchange in healthy men and women is comparable.

Women demonstrate small increases in both resting and exercise ventilation during pregnancy and the luteal phase of a menstrual cycle. This increase is attributable to of the rise in progesterone during pregnancy or the luteal phase of the menstrual cycle after ovulation. While this increase in ventilation during the luteal phase of the menstrual cycle might cause a modest loss of exercise

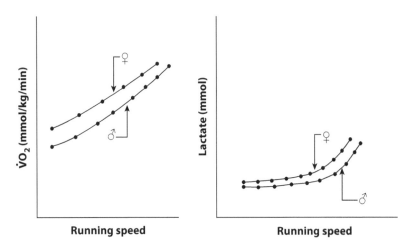

Figure 14.1 Difference between men and women on work economy during running, showing lean body weight corrected V̇O₂ (left graph) and serum lactate concentrations (right graph) at comparable percent of running speed.

efficiency, it does not impair athletic performance or produce an appreciable increase in dyspnea.

CARDIAC RESPONSE

For comparably sized subjects with any given workload, the heart rate in women is 5–10 beats/minute higher than in men. As size-adjusted stroke volume is similar in men and women, the higher heart rate likely reflects the requirement to perfuse the muscles with more volume because of the lower hemoglobin and arterial oxygen content in the blood of women. The systemic extraction of oxygen from arterial blood during a maximal exercise effort is not different, so that mixed venous oxygen content is not different between sexes. Because of hemoglobin concentration differences, for any given level of oxygen consumption, a woman will need to generate a higher cardiac output in comparison with a same-sized male (Figure 14.2).

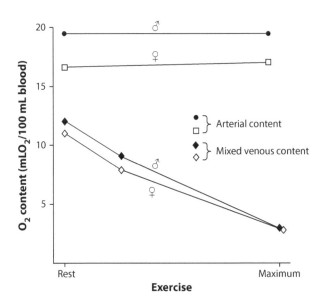

Figure 14.2 Changes in mixed venous oxygen content during a progressive work test in men (filled diamonds) and women (open diamonds). The lower arterial oxygen content in women (open squares) leads to a lower oxygen extraction in women despite comparable mixed venous content for both sexes.

SUMMARY

This chapter describes differences in the response to exercise between men and women. There are clearly more similarities than differences that make little difference in day-to-day life, but in spite of the increased participation and encouragement of women in competitive sports, clear gaps in race times and distances persist. There does appear to be a slight decrease in the economy of work, especially in running, in women, thus requiring a greater energy expenditure for work output. Although the ability to train the cardiopulmonary system and the peripheral tissues is similar, biomechanical differences, body composition, and pure strength are responsible for performance differences. The other issue is the lower hemoglobin level in women, requiring the heart to generate a higher cardiac output to maintain the same level of oxygen delivery.

15

Exercise testing the elderly

Appropriate interpretation of exercise test results on elderly patients is challenging for three different reasons: First, physiological changes that are medically classified as normal take place in the muscular, cardiovascular, and respiratory systems with aging, and these changes influence exercise findings.

Second, the most popular prediction equations for maximal oxygen uptake have not included subjects over 65 years old, and for smaller exercise data sets focusing on the elderly, there is a great deal of scatter such that age, for an over-65 population, becomes a relatively weak prediction factor. Finally, occult cardiovascular disease is more likely to be present in elderly subjects, so that making the distinction between normal aging physiology and early disease remains a diagnostic challenge.

This chapter discusses the following issues with exercise testing the elderly:

- Changes in exercising muscle
- Changes in cardiovascular function
- Changes in respiratory function
- Challenges with normal values and the influence of disease

CHANGES IN MUSCLE FIBER TYPE WITH NORMAL AGING

In every skeletal muscle, the proportion of fast-twitch or Type II fibers begins to decline progressively after age 30. While older subjects who remain physically active can minimize the loss of speed and power for two or even three decades, some fiber loss is relentless and cannot be prevented with training. Because the Type II fibers are the primary source of nonaerobic ATP production

from glycolysis, both lactate levels and metabolic acidosis are less during a maximal effort as the Type I (slow-twitch) fibers become the primary source of power for elderly subjects during a maximal effort.

The striking manifestation of this selective fiber type loss is that, during a CPET, the ventilatory threshold comes proportionately later during the test. Hence, for many healthy elderly subjects in their 80s, a ventilatory threshold may only be apparent near the final minute of a truly maximal effort.

MUSCLE MITOCHONDRIAL EFFICIENCY WITH AGING

By the sixth or seventh decade, all normal subjects will demonstrate some loss of mitochondrial efficiency. While the muscle mitochondria continue to consume oxygen and acetyl CoA to produce the hydrogen ion gradient that is needed to generate ATP from ADP, hydrogen ions can leak back across the inner mitochondrial membrane of an elderly subject, bypassing ATP synthetase, and thereby reduce ATP production despite the continued metabolism of oxygen and fuel. In the context of an exercise test, this means that the amount of oxygen required for a given power output will be higher. For example, a young subject cycling at 50 watts for several minutes and then increased to 100 watts will show an increase in oxygen consumption of around 500 cc O_2/minute at the higher load. An elderly subject will require nearly 600 cc O_2/minute to accomplish the same power output increase. If a progressive work protocol is conducted with an elderly subject using a very low watt increment, the same effect will be seen in the slope of the $\dot{V}O_2$/watt plot. A young

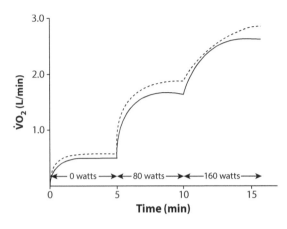

Figure 15.1 Oxygen consumption at 80 and 160 watt steady state workloads for a subject at age 55 (solid lines) and at age 75 (dotted lines).

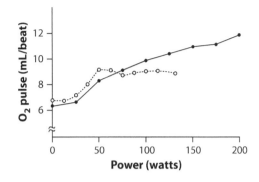

Figure 15.2 CPET O_2 pulse for a healthy 25-year-old woman (solid dots) and a healthy 75-year-old woman (open circles).

or middle-aged subject will have a slope of 10 cc O_2/watt, and an elderly subject will have a slope of 12–13 cc O_2/watt (Figure 15.1).

The end result of this effect is that an elderly subject requires a higher cardiac output and higher oxygen consumption to perform the same exercise task compared with the oxygen consumption requirements for that task in younger years. Hence, measurement of maximal oxygen uptake in elderly masters athletes modestly underestimates the actual loss of sustained exercise capacity with aging (as is documented by more obvious declines in race performance over time). While the loss of mitochondrial efficiency is seen in all elderly subjects, the effect is smaller in the chronically fit elderly and can be reduced in sedentary elderly subjects if they undergo aerobic training over a period of several months.

CARDIOVASCULAR SYSTEM CHANGES WITH NORMAL AGING

Diastolic dysfunction

Normal elderly subjects may demonstrate some degree of impaired ventricular diastolic filling that can be detected by echocardiography at rest, and this ventricular filling impairment further reduces the stroke volume with the higher heart rates of exercise. The normal progressive increase in O_2 pulse seen during a CPET depends on the combination of an unchanged exercise stroke volume

and the progressively increasing arterial-mixed venous O_2 content difference.

$$O_2 \text{ pulse} = (\dot{V}O_2/\text{Heart rate})$$
$$= (\text{Stroke volume})*(CaO_2 - CvO_2)$$

A normal elderly subject with mild diastolic dysfunction may demonstrate a modest reduction in stroke volume at higher heart rates. That reduction in stroke volume at higher heart rates will change the normal progression of the O_2 pulse during a CPET so that it will fail to continue to increase in the latter portion of the exercise effort (Figure 15.2).

Hence, at higher exercise heart rates, elderly subjects will have lower cardiac output and lower oxygen consumption in comparison with measurements made when they were younger. While mild diastolic dysfunction is generally said to be a consistent feature of normal aging, it is also present with nearly all myocardial diseases, and hence the distinction between normal aging and disease is often not clear. At least for aerobically fit elderly patients, the O_2 pulse plot usually increases in a near-normal fashion, suggesting that the age-related diastolic dysfunction is at least minimized by training.

Chronotropic impairment

Plots of maximal exercise heart rate versus age show an age-dependent decline in heart rate which appears linear. All of those data sets represent single measurements of exercised subjects encompassing a wide range of ages. However, longitudinal studies of maximal exercise heart rate in a few individuals have failed to show the regular reduction in maximal exercise heart rate suggested by the prediction equations. Just as age-predicted heart rates at any age reveal substantial normal variation, the same appears true for the reduction in maximal heart rate with aging. As noted in the section on cardiovascular disease, some element of exercise chronotropic impairment is a feature of all myocardial diseases, and this observation may contribute to the confusion as to appropriate normal values for maximal exercise heart rate in elderly subjects. Some healthy and chronically active elderly subjects can exceed age-predicted maximal exercise heart rates values by 20 or 30 beats/minute. For reductions in maximal exercise heart rate, as with diastolic dysfunction, the distinction between normal aging and significant chronotropic impairment is not always clear.

Delayed vascular recruitment

Blood flow to exercising muscles at the onset of exercise is delayed in elderly subjects. The normal vasodilation with exercise is nitric-oxide dependent and is especially reduced in sedentary elderly subjects. A common observation among elderly subjects is that even moderate levels of sustained exertion are more difficult in the first few minutes. Again, the extent of this impairment can be reduced with exercise training. The protocol used in a progressive work exercise test may be long enough to minimize this vascular recruitment exercise effect, but to our knowledge, whether or not this effect influences the CPET measurement $\dot{V}O_2$ max in the elderly has not been carefully investigated.

RESPIRATORY CHANGES WITH NORMAL AGING

Both vital capacity and FEV_1 slowly decline with normal aging, with more rapid decrease in the FEV_1, so that a normal FEV_1/FVC ratio of 82% in a subject in their mid-20s will reduce to less than 72% by their 70s. However, the effect of these age-related changes on maximal exercise ventilation in elderly patients without lung disease does not influence maximal exercise capacity. Just as with younger subjects, their minute ventilation at

maximal exercise will be well below their previously measured MVV. While the changes in spirometry with age are well-established and clearly related to aging effects on lung elasticity, there do not appear to be any age-related changes in pulmonary gas exchange during exercise in elderly subjects with normal lungs.

THE PROBLEM OF SELECTING APPROPRIATE NORMAL VALUES FOR THE ELDERLY

As noted, most of the maximal oxygen uptake measurements on populations have only included subjects under 65 years of age. Studies specifically focused on exercise in the elderly have generally used volunteers with a bias therefore toward the active. It does appear that maximal oxygen uptake in the healthy elderly is strongly influenced by a subject's life-long pattern of physical activity, leading to large differences between healthy active and healthy sedentary elderly subjects. For healthy nonobese elderly without functional limitations in activities of daily living, women over 65 years of age usually have a $\dot{V}O_2$ max in the 20–22 mL/kg/min range and men over 65 are in the 25–28 mL/kg/min range. For exceptionally active elderly subjects, increases above those values by 10–15 mL/kg/min should be expected.

THE CHALLENGE: DISTINGUISHING NORMAL AGEING FROM OCCULT DISEASE

As all of the aging-related exercise changes in elderly subjects described above progress very slowly, equivocal CPET abnormalities in an elderly subject who has experienced an appreciable loss of exercise tolerance over shorter periods of weeks or a few months merit further diagnostic exploration. For elderly subjects who present with new loss of exercise tolerance and no typical symptoms or ECG findings suggesting coronary disease, it is still prudent to consider exercise echocardiography as second test. While a CPET ECG finding of exercise-induced ischemia is relatively specific, the absence of ischemic exercise ECG changes in a CPET does not exclude coronary disease in a newly symptomatic elderly patient.

SUMMARY POINTS

- The proportion of fast-twitch muscle fibers decreases progressively with age. Beyond the loss of maximal muscle power, this change is manifested in elderly subjects during a CPET by a relatively late onset of arterial lactate and a late onset ventilatory threshold.
- Muscle mitochondria in elderly subjects develop a modest hydrogen ion leak from inner mitochondrial membranes. The exercise consequence of this aging effect is that increased oxygen consumption is required at a given level of aerobic work.
- Apparently healthy elderly subjects may demonstrate mild diastolic dysfunction, resulting in a lower exercise stroke volume and reduced maximal oxygen consumption. The relative severity of diastolic dysfunction appears to define the difference between normal aging and cardiac disease.

16

Exercise testing the obese

While the exercise limitation imposed by obesity is obvious, that limitation poses a challenge for the conduct and interpretation of diagnostic exercise testing. First, because an appropriate progressive work exercise protocol requires either ergometer or treadmill exercise, obese patients may face problems performing either mode, and modifications are required. Second, the onset of exercise for these patients requires a sudden substantial effort, and the effect of the sudden onset needs to be accounted for in the test interpretation. Finally, the interpretation of a maximal oxygen uptake measurement for an obese patient must be focused on the reason the test was requested.

- Selecting an appropriate exercise mode and protocol
- Effects of obesity on the initial exercise responses
- Interpreting the exercise test results

SELECTING AN APPROPRIATE EXERCISE MODE AND PROTOCOL

Just as for normal and overweight patients, a progressive work test for an obese patient must incorporate at least 50% of the muscle mass, so that either treadmill or ergometer exercise will be necessary. The choice between the two will be dictated by patient limitations. If the patient is able to sit and pedal on a cycle ergometer, the ergometer has the advantage of supporting the patient's weight, thereby providing a more gradual onset of exercise work load. Nevertheless, the thigh weight of an obese patient requires a substantial increase in oxygen uptake for simple unloaded pedaling. Depending on the size of the exercising thighs, the increase in oxygen consumption

in the transition from rest to unloaded pedaling may range between 400 and 600 mL/min. The watt increments chosen for the remainder of the protocol should be appropriate for an active normal subject of the same height. Otherwise healthy obese patients will have maximal oxygen consumptions somewhat above the height-predicted normal values.

If the obese patient is unable to sit and pedal on an ergometer, then treadmill exercise is the remaining option, and the treadmill protocol must be modified to take into account the very high oxygen cost of walking for obese patients. The figure below shows the progressive increase in oxygen consumption for a patient with a BMI of 45 whose treadmill protocol incorporated 0.5 mph increments per minute with zero grade. The oxygen cost of this protocol for an ideal body weight subject is shown as a dotted line (Figure 16.1).

As illustrated above, the substantial energy cost of moving a very large body on a treadmill is especially striking when compared with the cost for a normal-weight subject.

OBESITY AND INITIAL EXERCISE RESPONSES

For obese subjects with other underlying exercise limitations, the sudden increase in oxygen consumption with initiation of exercise may make it impossible to get the desired 8–10 minutes of exercise data for an optimal CPET study. The primary difficulty will be in identifying a ventilatory threshold, as that may even appear during the unloaded pedaling or the lowest treadmill walking speed. Nevertheless the maximal oxygen uptake

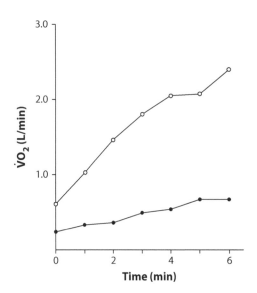

Figure 16.1 Oxygen consumption for a subject with a BMI of 45 (open circles) undergoing treadmill exercise at zero grade and 0.5 mph/minute exercise increments. Closed circles show exercise oxygen consumption for subject with same height and a BMI of 24 undergoing the same exercise protocol.

will still be a good representation of the maximal cardiac output.

A second consequence of the sudden increase in oxygen consumption with the initiation of exercise seen in some obese patients is transient oxygen desaturation in the first two minutes of exercise. Resolution of that oxygen desaturation as the exercise intensity increases is a normal finding. (A number of obese patients have been sent for diagnostic CPETs after they were observed to develop oxygen desaturation in the initial minute of a standard six-minute walk test.) For any normal BMI subject suddenly initiating heavy exercise (including running up stairs for normal-weight subjects), transient desaturation is a common finding. The physiology of this effect is that oxygen consumption at the muscle level goes up immediately with the onset of heavy exercise, leading to a rapid drop in the mixed venous oxygen saturation. The carbon dioxide produced within the exercising muscle is more soluble in tissues and takes longer to wash out, so the initial increase in exercise ventilation demonstrates an appreciable time lag relative to the increase in oxygen consumption measured at the mouth. The net effect is a transient drop in

alveolar and arterial PO_2, and if this sudden onset of heavy exercise in an obese patient is followed on a CPET exercise system, the respiratory R value ($\dot{V}CO_2/\dot{V}O_2$) will transiently drop well below 0.6 in association with the desaturation documented on the oximeter. If exercise can be sustained for more than three or four minutes, the arterial O_2 saturation and exercise R will return to normal exercise values.

INTERPRETING MAXIMAL OXYGEN UPTAKE IN OBESE SUBJECTS

The original rationale for normalizing maximal oxygen uptake by body mass was to simplify the test interpretation, when the intent was to compare exercise tolerance among subjects with a range of sizes. Obviously, normal large subjects would have larger maximal oxygen consumptions than small subjects, but the weight normalizations would make them comparable on a $\dot{V}O_2$-per-kilo basis. This normalization worked well in an era when obesity was relatively uncommon, but in our current era in which a majority of patients tested are overweight or obese, there are now two ways of considering that normalization. First, if the desire is to understand an obese patient's capacity to navigate the activities of daily living, they have to carry their increased body weight, and normalizing their measured maximal oxygen uptake by body weight provides a good index of their weight-related impairment to get around and accomplish physically demanding activities. If the goal of the exercise test is to obtain a surrogate estimate of maximal cardiac output, then weight normalization of that measurement is not appropriate. The appropriate choice for CPET evaluation of cardiac function in an obese patient is to compare the measurements acquired on the patient expressed in mL O_2/minute with the age, sex and height predicted normal values in mL O_2/minute. The expectation for maximal oxygen uptake for otherwise healthy overweight subjects is that their maximal oxygen uptake (in mL O_2/min) is roughly 10% higher than that of normal weight subjects of comparable height, sex, and age. That higher $\dot{V}O_2$ expectation likely represents the higher exercise requirements that obese patients must exert in activities of daily living.

SUMMARY POINTS

- Treadmill exercise testing for obese patients should incorporate very slow speeds and low grades in recognition of the very high oxygen demands of moving an obese body. Using only the standard protocol treadmill times to predict exercise oxygen consumption will very substantially underestimate an obese patient's true maximal oxygen consumption.
- Maximal oxygen uptake in obese patients should be compared to predicted normal values for patients of comparable age and height. Normalization of maximal oxygen consumption by weight will describe the level of functional impairment, but will underrepresent their maximal cardiac output.
- Obese patients may demonstrate transient desaturation within the initial two minutes of exercise during a six-minute walk or a CPET, and if that initial desaturation resolves as exercise progresses to higher levels of exertion, the finding is benign and requires no further evaluation.

17

Exercise testing elite aerobic athletes

For an individual to be able to perform in any sport at the national or international level, it takes an extraordinary combination of physiologic, psychologic, biomechanical, genetic, and biochemical characteristics, seasoned with good fortune, good support, and opportunity.

CHARACTERISTICS OF EXCEPTIONAL ATHLETES

- Muscular strength—training, genetic endowment
- Biomechanics—joint structure, training
- Coordination—genetic endowment, training
- Aerobic capacity—ventilation, cardiac output, oxygen extraction, training, genetic endowment
- Psychological—drive to train and win, coaching, opportunity

This chapter focuses on those athletes who need superb aerobic capacities to achieve success. This group sprints or endures but requires a cardiopulmonary engine to produce remarkable results. Additionally, the use of CPET to evaluate these athletes will be discussed.

HUMAN AEROBIC CAPACITY

Humans evolved into a bipedal machine that fit the "hunter-gatherer" lifestyle that insured survival. Evolving from a quadruped to a biped sacrificed speed but catered to the ability to cover great distances with stamina—the metered predator with evolving mental capacity to scheme success in the hunt. As humans in some parts of the world developed an agrarian society to supplement or supplant hunting, the ability to endure long periods of sustainable exertion was also beneficial.

The improvement of the human mental capacity, though, allowed for heterogeneity in physical abilities. Thus, the distribution of physical characteristics fell in a broad bell-shaped curve that still ensured reproduction and perpetuation of the species with less emphasis on physical capabilities. Humans could be tall, short, thin, fat, fast, or slow yet still endure, because within a populace, various skills could be employed to cover the contingencies of survival within the community; whereas, in the rest of the animal kingdom, the phenotypic expression of abilities fell in a much narrower bell-shaped curve. If a cheetah or antelope were slow or a mountain goat was clumsy, the animal would starve or be eaten or fall to its death. Humans had much more of a margin of safety because of broad skill sets, yet in the world of aerobic capacity, as one example of a survival strategy, humans are only modestly endowed as aerobic athletes. At one end of the human bell-shaped curve though are those people who have exceptional aerobic capabilities, which afford them the opportunities to excel in either the world where physical stress imposes potential barriers for survival or in the athletic arena where these attributes contribute to success.

This chapter describes some of the known inherited or acquired skills that contribute to athletic success but will not deal extensively with the effects of training, which will be discussed in Chapter 18.

ELITE AEROBIC CAPACITY

Although a high aerobic capacity ($\dot{V}O_2$ max) alone is not enough to get one to win endurance events in championship competitions, it is one of the major factors without which an athlete must have modest, more recreational goals. In a group of healthy subjects in their 20s or 30s, the average $\dot{V}O_2$ max ranges from the mid-30s to mid-40s mL/kg/min. Exceptional aerobic athletes, such as middle- and long-distance runners, cyclists, cross-country skiers, or rowers may have values of $\dot{V}O_2$ max in the 70–85 mL/kg/min range. Sprinters and field and court athletes have their own exceptional characteristics, but their $\dot{V}O_2$ max values are usually somewhere between the endurance athletes and normal values (Figure 17.1). No amount of training can elevate a normal person to the extraordinary capability to generate energy as the elite athletes. What parts of the oxygen delivery and utilization process is different in these people?

To put human performance in perspective with other individuals in the animal kingdom, consider measurements made in dogs, thoroughbred race horses, and pronghorn antelopes. Those three species of exceptional aerobic animals have values of $\dot{V}O_2$ max of approximately 125, 150, and 300 mL/kg/minute, respectively. The antelope, especially, relies on the ability to maintain exercise for prolonged periods of time at a high percentage of their $\dot{V}O_2$ max to stay out of the reach of predators, while the racehorse was engineered by breeders a few hundred years ago to have extraordinary performance over a couple of minutes.

Cardiac

The major physiologic advantage that characterizes highly accomplished aerobic athletes is a high maximal exercise cardiac output. The ability to generate large volumes of blood flow during high levels of work (35–42 L/min in male athletes) is a function of a large stroke volume, vascular compliance, and rapid end-diastolic filling. This capacity is largely inherited but also has a component of trainability. Whereas maximum heart rate is not different in elite athletes, and is not changed with training, resting heart rates may be as low as 30 beats/minute, providing an exceptionally high heart rate range (maximal exercise HR–resting HR) compared with normal subjects. As resting cardiac output is not different in elite athletes, this low resting heart rate is simply a consequence of a very large stroke volume. The oxygen pulse attained at the end of a CPET is proportional to the stroke volume and may exceed values of 30 mL/beat in large elite athletes. While exercise stroke volume in normal subjects remains unchanged after the initiation of ergometer

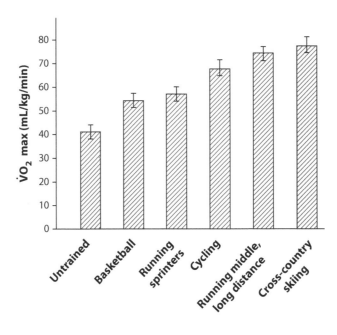

Figure 17.1 Examples of maximum oxygen consumptions ($\dot{V}O_2$ max, mL/kg/min) in humans from healthy normal nonathletes, as well as accomplished aerobic athletes from several types of sporting events.

or treadmill exercise, stroke volume in elite aerobic athletes may show a modest progressive increase at the highest tolerated exertional levels. The mechanism responsible for this increase is unknown.

Another cardiac characteristic associated with high levels of aerobic training is resting heart rate variability (HRV). HRV is thought to reflect a well-trained heart and occurs with increasing parasympathetic tone incurred with training. In contrast, individuals with little to no resting HRV have a higher incidence of adverse cardiac events.

Ventilation and gas exchange

While successful aerobic athletes tend to have modestly increased vital capacities compared with normal subjects, a striking difference is observed among elite swimmers, who show average vital capacities of 120% of age- and height-predicted values. As swimming is the only sport in which breathing is restricted, a larger lung volume enables both a lower breathing rate and better buoyancy. While adults cannot increase their vital capacity with training, studies of children who have trained as swimmers during their preadolescent growth suggest that they have greater gains in lung volumes compared with active children who were not training as swimmers.

Competitive aerobic athletes, in general, show a lower ventilatory response during exercise. During a CPET, this manifests as a low ventilatory equivalent for oxygen ($\dot{V}E/\dot{V}O_2$) during submaximal exercise. As described earlier, a normal $\dot{V}E/\dot{V}O_2$ at rest and during sustainable work is in the mid-to-high 20 liters/min range, while some endurance runners or cyclists will have values as low as 16–18 liters/min. With that relatively lower exercise ventilation, these athletes will have lower work of breathing and relatively elevated end-tidal CO_2 readings in comparison with normal subjects.

While the relatively low exercise ventilation that is characteristic of the average endurance athlete leads to modestly lower values of alveolar O_2 during exercise and higher alveolar levels of CO_2, a subset of elite endurance athletes may demonstrate moderate arterial hypoxemia during heavy exercise. In these athletes with very high exercise cardiac outputs, the residence time for blood in the alveolar capillaries is too short to allow full oxygenation, creating a true diffusion limitation for oxygen uptake at sea level.

Peripheral extraction

The advantages of the elite aerobic athlete continues in the extraction and utilization of oxygen and fuel sources, part of which is inherited and part of which is trained. To optimize oxygen delivery, the body must supply even blood flow at the microvascular level. Training improves microvascular blood flow, mediated by a number of biochemical factors resulting in an increase in nitric oxide (NO). There is growing evidence that elite aerobic athletes have some genetic differences with angiotensin-converting enzyme-1 (ACE-1) that can perpetrate improvement in blood flow. A large portion of high-level sprinters are endowed with a skeletal muscle actin-binding protein (alpha-actin-3) that appears to facilitate fast-twitch muscle function.

In addition to the higher delivery of oxygenated blood to the exercising muscle groups, the trained muscle groups of elite athletes effectively have facilitated diffusion of oxygen from the blood to the mitochondria as a consequence of increased capillary density and increased mitochondrial density in muscles that have been trained continuously over a sustained period of time. The net effect of this improved muscle oxygen extraction can lead to mixed venous oxygen extraction of over 80% in highly trained athletes.

Muscle cell fiber type

There are two basic muscle fiber types, slow twitch (Type I) and fast twitch (Type II), the latter of which is further categorized as Type IIa and IIb. Whereas, the "twitch" term denotes literal contraction and function, the designations of Type I, Type IIa, and IIb convey important differences in fuel utilization and metabolic function. Type I fibers are mitochondrially dense and thus highly oxidative, utilizing largely free fatty acids (FFA) as a major fuel source; whereas, Type II fibers are glycogen rich, which, when activated, rely primarily on glucose metabolism and glycolysis for fuel and energy generation. Type II cells are the primary site of anaerobic metabolism during maximal effort. Type IIa fibers exhibit plasticity with training and can become more aerobic in their function.

Among humans, there is a wide spectrum in the distribution of fiber types; whereas, other animals, based on their need for function and thus survival, have a narrower spectrum. In a large normal population of humans, the distribution of muscle fiber type in muscles of locomotion is approximately 55% Type I and 45% Type II. Numerous studies though have shown that athletes who are outstanding endurance athletes may have 80%–90% Type I fibers. Likewise, outstanding sprinters and power athletes will have a predominance of Type II fibers. These fiber-type distributions appear to be genetically determined, although with endurance training, Type IIa cells can actually transform to functional Type I fibers. There does not appear to be any intervention that will increase the proportion of Type II cells in a Type I athlete.

The importance of the metabolic transformation of Type IIa cells is that the body, by both inheritance and training, can much more efficiently utilize FFAs at higher levels of work before having to lapse into glycolysis, which limits heavy exercise duration in comparison to FFA utilization.

This adaptation from an evolutionary and survival perspective is obviously beneficial, for the individual who can exert at a higher level of sustainable work can run from a predator or run after prey longer and faster.

Understanding these concepts has important implications while using CPET to evaluate athletes on a longitudinal basis. Not only can $\dot{V}O_2$ max be tracked but so can the ventilatory or lactate threshold, as landmarks for both training and fuel utilization.

SUMMARY

This chapter has described some of the characteristics that are characteristic of a highly accomplished aerobic athlete. It has focused on the elements that optimize oxygen delivery and utilization—cardiopulmonary and muscular attributes that operate on the same principles as "normal" individuals but at a higher level.

Characteristics of elite aerobic athletes

1. Superior $\dot{V}O_2$ max, much of which is inherited and some trained

2. Pulmonary: modestly higher lung volumes and normal gas exchange in most circumstances
3. Cardiac: higher exercise cardiac output secondary to a genetically determined large stroke volume, further improved by training
4. Muscle fiber type characteristics inherited, with local muscle training adaptations in microcirculation, mitochondrial density and fuel utilization in Type IIa fibers

18

Exercise training: The role of CPET

This chapter describes the role of CPET in evaluating training responses in patients, athletes, and normal individuals. It is not within the purview of this chapter to undertake an exhaustive review of the complex mechanisms at work when an individual initiates a sustained increase in physical activity. However, we will review the effects of training that can be documented objectively with CPET testing. We define fitness attained through training as an ability to sustain a higher level of work for a longer period of time.

In almost all states of health and disease, an individual can improve physical functioning by a program of training that, at the very least, will result in better daily functioning. CPET testing provides objective documentation of changes in aerobic fitness that are useful both for the patient or athletes in consultation with the health care team or coaching staff. This chapter will describe the insights that CPET can provide in documenting progress in patients' physical rehabilitation or athletes' training.

The following topics will be described:

- Overview
- Training for everyone
- Aerobic fitness (peak performance, $\dot{V}O_2$ max)
- Sustainable work and endurance—ventilatory/anaerobic threshold
- Fuel utilization—metabolic effect
- Pulmonary function
- Peripheral adaptation—muscle cell and capillaries
- Genetic influence
- Deconditioning
- Overtraining syndrome

OVERVIEW

Improving aerobic fitness necessarily involves the use of the body's large muscles. The consequence is not only an improvement in cardiopulmonary health but also in muscle strength and stability. Thus, one's function in daily life or competitive performance is improved on a number of levels. This improvement is particularly important in older patients, both healthy individuals as well as those with heart and lung disease, in whom balance and strength are declining and in whom improved strength and endurance may prevent falls and injury. Aerobic training will improve muscle strength, joint mobility, and neuromuscular function. Strength training is equally important for older subjects, but that topic will not be addressed here.

A basic concept of aerobic training is that, to achieve a training affect, an individual must undertake a training load of

- Adequate intensity
- Sufficient duration
- Consistent frequency

to result in measurable differences that translate into improved function.

SUBJECTS

Unless there are severe neurologic, orthopedic, or cardiopulmonary limitations, all individuals can improve physical performance. It is, therefore, important for the clinician, the therapist, or the coach to be able to understand how best to advise their subjects so that activities of daily living or athletic performance can be improved. The ability of an individual with heart or lung disease to once again be able to take a nightly walk with a friend or a spouse to retrieve mail each day is just as important as climbing Mount Everest or winning a sports medal.

The principles of training for each of these groups are identical; it is only a matter of degree that separates the well person from a patient on the one hand or an athlete on the other. The physical therapist, the advising clinician, and the athletic trainer or coach must all be aware of the same physiologic effects that an increase in an exercise program will convey on their subjects.

For instance, an endurance athlete may undertake an intense program of both aerobic and interval training to reach a level of performance that may take months or years to attain. Or a patient may undergo a supervised program of both strength and aerobic training 3–4 times a week for a number of weeks to simply achieve improved everyday performance and well-being.

AEROBIC FITNESS

The gold standard for the measurement of one's peak aerobic fitness is maximum oxygen consumption ($\dot{V}O_2$ max). Its measurement is well described in several areas of this book, and reproducible measurements from CPET testing are critical in tracking progress. Although an important marker, $\dot{V}O_2$ max must be taken in context with other variables which sometimes have more important implications for sustained performance.

$\dot{V}O_2$ max improves with concerted aerobic training. The degree of improvement, however, is quite variable, based in large part on the training program as well as the individual's genetic characteristics. It is generally accepted that most sedentary subjects will attain roughly a 15% improvement in $\dot{V}O_2$ max after a training program of a few months, but there is appreciable variability in response that may range between 0%–30%. There appears to be a heritable trait that determines the extent of possible training response. Nevertheless, while a healthy 30-year old with a $\dot{V}O_2$ max in the low 40 mL/kg/min range can become more fit, he could never attain the $\dot{V}O_2$ max of an elite aerobic athlete capable of 70–85 mL/kg/min.

Adequate aerobic training involves a regular program of exertion, working utilizing at least 50% of maximum output, and exercising several times a week for at least 30 minutes each session. Other types of training are discussed later. Some of the outcomes of aerobic training will be briefly outlined.

Cardiac

First, with sustained training there is an increase in both plasma volume and red cell mass, with a slightly greater increase in plasma volume, so that hemoglobin concentration may decrease slightly over time. This combination of responses in the circulating blood volume results in an increase in oxygen delivery that is secondary both to an increase in cardiac output as well as oxygen-carrying capacity.

Cardiac adaptation is one of the most critical events in aerobic training. Like any muscle, the heart adapts to a consistent increase in training activity by an increase in stroke volume. Highly trained endurance athletes have been found to have total stroke volumes 15%–25% larger than sedentary size-matched controls, with at least some of this increased size attributable to the training regimen.

With training, there is an increase ventricular compliance permitting more rapid filling during diastole, larger end-diastolic volumes, and improved ventricular contractility, all contributing to an increased stroke volume. Adaptations to training within the myocardium are similar to those of striated muscle, with an increase in capillary density resulting in improved perfusion.

All of these changes—increased blood volume, myocardial contractility and strength, myocardial perfusion—result in lower heart rates at rest and submaximal exercise levels; whereas, *maximum exercise heart rate does not change* with training. The change in the total chronotropic range with training is most likely an autonomically mediated response to the improved stroke volume. Thus, a major contributor to the improvement in aerobic capacity comes from an increase in maximum cardiac output. This finding is readily suggested during a standard CPET by an increase in maximal oxygen uptake (Figure 18.1).

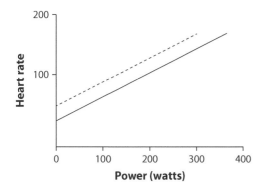

Figure 18.1 The effect of aerobic training on heart rate from resting to maximum workloads showing lower resting and submaximum heart rates at comparable work intensities after training (solid line) compared with the untrained state (dashed line). Maximum heart rates do not change. These findings are a result of the development of a larger stroke volume with training.

SUSTAINABLE WORK AND ENDURANCE

Because daily activity does not usually involve repeated bouts of maximum work, a practical outcome of training is the enhancement of the intensity of exertion that one can sustain for prolonged periods of time. This change is important not only for competitive athletes but also active normal individuals and patients with heart and lung disease. As has been described on a number of occasions in this book, the point above which one cannot maintain a given intensity of work for more than a few minutes is called the ventilatory, lactate, or anaerobic threshold (V_T, AT.) Aerobic training will result in the V_T occurring at a higher percentage of the total CPET time.

Thus, an individual can sustain a higher level of exertion that is greater in the trained than in the untrained state. The athlete can sustain a faster pace; the patient can perform daily activities and recreation more productively.

A great deal of research has been done about the plasticity of the V_T, the marker for determining the maximal point where sustainable work can be continued. Early studies showed that intensive training improved the V_T 44%, expressed as absolute value, and 15% as expressed relative to the $\dot{V}O_2$ max. Numerous studies have looked at the volume and type of training that results in optimal improvement of $\dot{V}O_2$ max and V_T.

Interval training

Researchers have transferred methods that have been used in training for many years to the laboratory and began to look at interval training (IT) as a supplement to aerobic training. IT has many forms and configurations but is basically described as a series of intense bouts above the V_T interspersed with recovery periods. Usually middle distance and endurance athletes will do some level of endurance training every day and then add IT 2–3 days per week. It was thought that very intense exercise levels signal greater changes in the muscle oxidative capacity that otherwise would not be stimulated by endurance training. Studies have used various lengths of time of intense exercise from 20 seconds to four minutes, with a comparable spread in the recovery periods. The important findings have been that there has been some improvement in $\dot{V}O_2$ max but more importantly a movement of the V_T to higher levels of exertion even with very short bouts of high exertion in IT training. As would be expected, with training the onset of increases in serum lactate follow the later V_T.

From a practical standpoint for healthy individuals, interval training can be introduced easily while walking, running, or cycling. The subject will maintain a sustainable pace with timed bouts of high exertion to tolerance followed by a recovery after which a repeat bout of intense exertion can be undertaken. The subject may start out with just one period of intense exercise for a few training sessions and then increase the number of those bouts gradually to a point where 6–10 intense bouts can be undertaken. Patients can also be supervised with care to a modified form of IT training depending on the underlying severity of their disease.

FUEL UTILIZATION

Training has an effect on the fuel utilization for energy that plays an important role in the beneficial shift of the V_T. The three primary muscle fuel sources are carbohydrates (including muscle glycogen), free fatty acids (FFA), and a very small contribution from proteins during very prolonged exercise. The body has far more energy available as FFA and much smaller amounts of glycogen in muscle or liver. The fuel that is utilized depends on

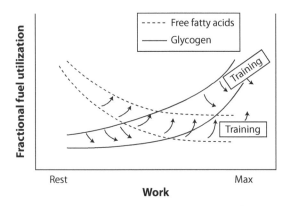

Figure 18.2 The effect of aerobic training on fuel utilization during exercise showing that free fatty acids (FFA, dashed lines) are the primary fuel during sustainable levels of work; whereas, at work intensities above the ventilatory threshold, glycogen (solid lines) is the primary fuel. Aerobic training results in a shift in fuel utilization such that FFAs supply a greater fraction of fuel at any given level of work.

the intensity of exercise, and training has an effect on allocation of those fuels (Figure 18.2).

For sustainable levels of exercise, the primary fuels are fat and carbohydrate. As one gets near exhaustive levels of work, glycogen is broken down by glycolysis and is used as a fuel source. The determination of fuel use is determined by:

1. Type of exercise—light or heavy, short or prolonged, sustained or intermittent
2. Level of training
3. Dietary intake

The relative proportion of fats and carbohydrates utilized in light and moderate exercise is reflected by the respiratory exchange ratio (R, $\dot{V}CO_2/\dot{V}O_2$) at rest and during exercise. During a CPET, the respiratory R is always displayed. However, after the onset of the ventilatory threshold, the additional contribution of CO_2 from hyperventilation obscures that measurement as a marker of proportionate metabolic fuel use.

The use of fuels during exercise is appropriately distributed based on their availability. In a resting state and at lower levels of sustainable work, carbohydrate and fat contribute equally. At a sustainable level of work for several hours, a greater proportion of the energy source is derived from fat as the contribution of carbohydrate decreases.

On the other hand, as the intensity of exercise increases, carbohydrates become the more important fuel source. At near maximal levels of work, glycogen becomes the principal source of fuel as oxygen delivery becomes inadequate for the exercise demand. At lower levels of work, the ready availability of oxygen to exercising muscle facilitates FFA use.

Training does shift the pattern of fuel utilization in a way that makes inherent sense for function and survival. As aerobic fitness increases and oxygen availability is augmented, FFAs are used at higher intensities of work, and glycogen utilization is minimized. This phenomenon is reflected in the lower levels of lactate after training above the V_T and at $\dot{V}O_2$ max. This shift in fuel utilization is important for sustained exercise because there are far larger FFA sources within muscle and from blood compared with muscle glycogen stores. When the laws of nature dictate survival of the fittest, the creature that can run the longest with adequate fuel supply will neither starve nor be eaten (Figure 18.3).

PULMONARY FUNCTION

The mechanical function of breathing sustains an adequate balance of oxygen and carbon dioxide in the arterial blood throughout exercise. It is thus curious that physical training results in minimal anatomic or physiologic pulmonary adaptations. For instance, gas exchange and airflow are not affected by training, although there are some

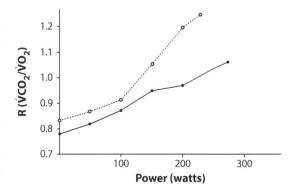

Figure 18.3 Comparison of the respiratory R during a CPET for a subject in a marathon-trained state (solid dots) and four years later, without training (open circles).

modest respiratory muscle adaptations that may contribute to improved exercise performance.

First, it is important to recognize that breathing takes work. The muscles of respiration consume oxygen just like any other muscle, and the so-called work of breathing increases progressively with higher levels of ventilation. Breathing consumes approximately 3% of resting metabolic rate, whereas, at maximal exercise in a normal individual, work of breathing may consume nearly 10% of energy expenditure. Training does not improve respiratory efficiency in normal individuals. It seems counterintuitive from an evolutionary standpoint that while the muscles of locomotion to flee or pursue need a greater supply of oxygen to go faster, the work of breathing is "stealing" some of the cardiac output that otherwise could go to the legs.

In contrast to normal subjects, patients with pulmonary diseases have increased resistive and/or elastic loads to breathing that may make the work of breathing during exercise totally incapacitating for the patient.

Dyspnea is one of the most cogent symptoms that causes an individual to stop exercising. The more inefficient that lung mechanics become, the greater the dyspnea. Athletes, who tend to experience less severe dyspnea with exercise, show a respiratory pattern with relatively larger tidal volumes and lower respiratory rates, possibly secondary to sustained training experience. Exercise ventilatory equivalents for both oxygen and carbon dioxide tend to be lower in athletes, possibly a result of both efficient lung mechanics as well as lower exercise respiratory drives. Thus, on a CPET, both $\dot{V}E/\dot{V}O_2$ and $\dot{V}E/\dot{V}CO_2$ tend to be lower for well-trained subjects.

Patients with both obstructive and restrictive lung disease have a number of factors that have been described in other chapters that result in a greater work of breathing and dyspnea. Several techniques are used in pulmonary rehabilitation programs to improve respiratory muscle strength and efficiency that decrease dyspnea and the $\dot{V}E/\dot{V}O_2$ and $\dot{V}E/\dot{V}CO_2$. For instance, resistive training of the respiratory muscles can improve inspiratory muscle strength and endurance and enhance daily function.

PERIPHERAL ADAPTATIONS

Whole body aerobic training by its nature involves the use of large muscle mass. With a large increase in cardiac output during heavy exercise, the involved muscles must be accurately allocated appropriate proportions of total blood flow. The capacitance of the arterial system, especially to the large leg muscles, far outstrips the human heart's ability to fill those vessels. Thus, the autonomic nervous system must balance vasoconstriction and vasodilatation to optimize blood flow and oxygen delivery to the exercising muscles while still preserving adequate blood pressure for coronary and cerebral perfusion.

While the discussion of the increases in maximal oxygen uptake with training thus far has focused on cardiac and hematologic adaptations, maximal oxygen uptake will also be increased if there is enhanced peripheral extraction within the exercising muscle groups. The Fick equation depicts the oxygen extraction contribution to oxygen uptake as the arterial-to-mixed venous oxygen content difference $(CaO_2 - CvO_2)$. As measurement of this difference requires either a pulmonary artery catheter to sample mixed venous blood or measurements of exercise cardiac output, it is not part of a standard CPET. Nevertheless, the extent of oxygen extraction at maximal effort is an important component of the overall maximal oxygen uptake. Both normal subjects and cardiac patients giving a maximal effort will ordinarily extract about 75% of the arterial oxygen content.

Some component of the training response to maximal exercise performance includes the slow adaptation of the trained muscle groups to enhance oxygen extraction from the arterial blood. Capillary delivery of oxygenated blood is certainly crucial, but the oxygen still must diffuse through muscle tissue to the muscle mitochondria to support ATP production. Sustained intense training of muscle groups over many months results in increased muscle mitochondrial content, increased muscle myoglobin, and increased muscle capillary density, factors that effectively improve the diffusion limitation for oxygen moving from capillary lumen to mitochondrial matrix. Note that these adaptations, unlike the cardiac and hematologic adaptations, are specific to the muscles involved in the training. Because measurements to confirm this improved peripheral extraction of oxygen require femoral venous catheters and/or pulmonary artery catheters, the relative importance of these muscle changes to increase maximal oxygen uptake is not well quantitated. However, mixed venous oxygen saturations well below 20% with maximal effort have been documented in well-trained aerobic athletes, in contrast to the 25%–30% saturations ordinarily observed in normal subjects with maximal effort.

GENETIC INFLUENCES

As mentioned earlier, the measurement of $\dot{V}O_2$ max within any individual is a reproducible variable that is a hallmark variable of CPET. But the degree of improvement between individuals, regardless of high levels of training, is quite variable. Five months of supervised aerobic training in previously sedentary adults resulted in a mean improvement in $\dot{V}O_2$ max of over 15%, but with a substantial range of improvement between 0%–30%. The extent of improvement was linked within families, so that there clearly exists a heritability of trainability. Thus, if one is using CPET to track an athlete's or a patient's improvement in fitness, one must remember that $\dot{V}O_2$ max will ordinarily improve to a variable extent, but that the metabolic changes in exercise fuel utilization manifested by the ventilatory threshold are equally as important to monitor and useful for encouragement.

DECONDITIONING

Understanding deconditioning is just as important as understanding training.

Deconditioning will be defined as the decrease in aerobic conditioning and muscular strength that occurs with chosen or imposed immobilization.

Periods of inactivity lead to a decrease in aerobic conditioning and muscular strength and result in an increase in morbidity and a decrease in quality of life. It is thus equally important for the practitioner, coach, trainer, or therapist to understand how an individual can lose fitness from illness, injury, or choice and therefore try to minimize that loss, as well as recoup it in recovery. In this section, we will deal primarily with aerobic fitness in the use of CPET in tracking its regression or progress.

A number of studies have documented the effect of imposed sedentary conditions, such as bed rest, on peak aerobic capacity. Those classic studies have shown that 20 days or more of bed rest result in almost a 30% decrease in $\dot{V}O_2$ max for fit subjects and somewhat smaller reduction for sedentary

subjects. The decrease in peak $\dot{V}O_2$ was proportional to the duration of bed rest. The onset of the V_T or lactate threshold also came at an earlier percentage of $\dot{V}O_2$ max on a progressive exercise test. Maximal exercise heart rate was unchanged with the reduction in $\dot{V}O_2$ max, suggesting an inactivity-related reduction in stroke volume, also manifested as a higher heart rate at any given work load. In summary, the decrease in aerobic function with sustained sedentary state is almost a mirror image of all of the aforementioned processes of improvement during training.

Muscle atrophy also begins very early with complete immobilization, such as when a broken limb is put in a cast. However, bed rest alone also contributes to muscle atrophy over time, albeit in a less dramatic fashion. It is important to understand that all of these decrements can be reversed with a program of aerobic and strength training. This concept is equally as important in the patient with COPD or a patient with a prolonged surgical recovery as it is in a competitive athlete. CPET testing is a very useful tool to document the degree of decrease or increase in aerobic capacity both for the clinician as well as the coach because it can provide objective data that may provide incentive to the athlete or patient.

OVER-TRAINING SYNDROME

Improvement in athletic performance requires a careful orchestration of workloads of progressive intensity to a peak level. The level of intensity is usually limited by prudent coaches or tolerance from the athlete. However, there are many top-flight athletes who push themselves to such a degree that the level of peak aerobic fitness drops, sometimes to a severe degree. These are often athletes who are so obsessed with training that they have no other life, so they adapt a training philosophy that more is better and may incur "over-training syndrome (OTS)."

These athletes, more often aerobic athletes, are referred for medical evaluation when their training or competitive performance is noticeably worse, with slower times. However, before considering over-training as a diagnosis, it is crucial for the clinician to exclude an underlying illness that is affecting performance. Elite athletes with small, recurrent pulmonary emboli, for example may still be capable of maximal oxygen uptakes well above normal values. A thorough history and physical should be performed and appropriate laboratory tests sent. Talking with the athlete about his/her lifestyle, social life, and training routines is critical. Entities that can begin in a subtle manner that can mimic OTS include iron deficiency; EBV or other viral, bacterial, or fungal infections; POTS; depression; and leukemias and other malignancies.

When an appropriate medical work-up is unrevealing and the training history is consistent with the OTS, then it is reasonable to perform a CPET. There usually is not a baseline test, but one can estimate what the $\dot{V}O_2$ max and V_T should be based on the sport and peak performance of the athlete, and a relative reduction in the $\dot{V}O_2$ max is ordinarily evident. If the $\dot{V}O_2$ max and history support OTS, then the difficult task is to convince the athlete, his coaches, friends, and family that, to get over OTS, it is critical to cut back training drastically for an indeterminate but prolonged period of time. This advice is a death knell for most of these athletes who will often not heed the advice and continue to train, or feign laying off while sneaking off to train surreptitiously. In this behavioral aspect, these noncompliant individuals share characteristics with anorexia nervosa patients. With compliance and a drastically reduced training schedule, OTS resolves and the athlete can return to training and eventually competing at their peak level. CPET, if performed at propitious times during the course of the syndrome, can be a useful tool to document recovery where $\dot{V}O_2$ max and V_T will improve.

The etiology of OTS is not known. Intense training with inadequate time for recovery between intervals, training sessions, or competition is the *sine qua non*, but the understanding of what is involved in recovery is not forthcoming. Neuromuscular, immune, autonomic nervous system, metabolic, psychological, and endocrine overload and their complex interactions have been postulated as etiologic factors, but no clear mechanism for OTS has been discovered. As it stands, it is a clinical diagnosis that requires belief in its existence and prolonged support for the athlete who will get better without any therapy other than time and encouragement.

SUMMARY

This chapter addresses the topic of training of the aerobic capacity of patients, athletes, and normal individuals. It emphasizes the various physiologic components that are involved in an individual's improvement in function and performance, as well as the use of CPET as an ideal tool to monitor improvement. Additionally, an important message is that improved function is practically demonstrated by an individual's ability to carry on a task more efficiently and faster for a longer period of time. Thus, $\dot{V}O_2$ max is only a part of the evaluation of training; whereas, sustainable work is better monitored by later appearance of the ventilatory threshold in a CPET effort.

19

Cardiac and pulmonary rehabilitation

Both cardiac and pulmonary rehabilitation programs have demonstrated important benefits and improved outcomes for participating patients. Both of these disease-oriented programs include an exercise training component, but it is important to recognize that all effective rehabilitation programs include many other important elements beyond exercise training that contribute to their demonstrated efficacy. The limited focus of this chapter, however, is to describe the use of a standard CPET to choose appropriate individual exercise training levels for the patients who plan to participate in these programs.

EXERCISE TRAINING IN CARDIAC REHABILITATION

The clinical benefits of exercise training were first identified in patients with ischemic heart disease and subsequently have been established in both heart failure with reduced ejection fraction and heart failure with preserved ejection fraction. More recently, positive post-training outcomes have been identified even for patients with idiopathic pulmonary hypertension, with the caveat that all of these patients undergoing training had already been optimally stabilized on appropriate pulmonary hypertension treatments.

Prior to beginning the formal exercise training portion of a cardiac rehabilitation program, the patient must be clinically stable and on fixed medically appropriate treatment. For a majority of cardiac patients, this includes some level of beta blockade, and for patients with severe systolic heart failure, implanted defibrillators. The performance of a standard CPET before beginning the aerobic exercise portion of a cardiac rehabilitation program includes the benefit of being able to identify

inappropriate hypotension, exercise-associated arrhythmias, or ischemic changes before starting the program. However, the primary rationale is to identify the appropriate training load to be applied to the patient based on the heart rate during treadmill or ergometer exercise.

The aerobic portion of most cardiac rehabilitation programs will last 12 weeks, including at least three exercise bouts per week. The duration of aerobic training may start at 15–20 minutes and progress, as tolerated, to 35–40 minutes. The intensity of exercise chosen is based on the heart rate achieved at some given treadmill speed and grade or ergometer watt load. As was described in previous chapters, the exercise heart rate is directly linked to the level of exertion, so that the most convenient means of monitoring the intensity of an exercise training stimulus is to identify an individual goal exercise heart rate. The intensity goal for most programs is to have the patient work at 60% of their maximal exercise capacity, although some programs will eventually work up to 70%, or even 80%, of maximal exercise capacity. Identifying the appropriate exercise heart rate for that 60% goal makes use of the calculation of heart rate reserve.

Heart rate reserve (HRR)
= Maximal exercise heart rate − Resting heart rate

For an exercise intensity that is 60% of maximum, the desired heart rate is

$$\text{Training heart rate} = 0.6 \times (\text{HRR}) + \text{Resting heart rate}$$

For example, a 60% exercise stimulus for a 45-year-old heart-failure patient, with a resting heart rate of 60 and a maximal heart rate of 120, would have a 60% exertional heart rate of

$$\text{Training heart rate} = 0.6 \times (120 - 60) + 60$$
$$= 96 \text{ beats/min}$$

The use of an age-predicted maximal heart rate to determine the training stimulus is especially inappropriate for patients with underlying heart disease, given both the chronotropic limitation of most myocardial diseases and the clinical benefits of drugs with beta-blocking effects. Simply multiplying the normal predicted heart rate by desired percent of maximal exercise intensity, as suggested in some publications, also ignores the role of the resting heart rate. Doing the latter calculation for the patient described above, where heart rate range was based on CPET measurements, using an assumed maximal heart rate (220 − age) gives the following training heart rate:

$$\text{Training heart rate} = 0.6 \times (220 - 45)$$
$$= 105 \text{ beats/min}$$

TRAINING-ASSOCIATED EXERCISE CHANGES IN CARDIAC REHAB PATIENTS

Clinical trials of cardiac rehabilitation programs have demonstrated mild improvements in maximal oxygen uptake, with increases in stroke volume and reduction in resting heart rate. The neurohumeral markers of heart failure are reduced, as suggested by a reduction in ventilatory equivalent for CO_2. In addition, the markers for inflammation that are increased in cardiac disease appear to be reduced by exercise training.

EXERCISE TRAINING IN PULMONARY REHABILITATION

COPD patients completing a pulmonary rehabilitation program have improved submaximal exercise tolerance and show a significant reduction in the risk for COPD exacerbation. As noted in the obstructive diseases chapter, standard CPETs are not ordinarily performed on COPD patients, but for patients under consideration for a pulmonary rehabilitation program, a preliminary test offers useful information. First, as the majority of COPD patients are former smokers, they have a significant incidence of unsuspected coronary artery disease that may be revealed during a standard CPET. Second, the exercise intensity that a COPD patient can sustain is poorly predicted by the extent of their airflow obstruction. Hence, a standard CPET allows assessment of an appropriate power output to choose to attain a training effect.

CONDUCT OF A CPET FOR PATIENTS REQUIRING SUPPLEMENTAL OXYGEN

An appreciable number of COPD patients sent for pulmonary rehabilitation require supplemental oxygen during exercise, and they must be exercised while breathing supplemental oxygen for their pretraining CPET. Because a mask or mouthpiece is required to monitor ventilation, the simplest supplemental oxygen administration approach is to connect a bag containing 30% oxygen to a two-way non-rebreathing Hans Rudolph valve. (Note that the CPET system gas and ventilation sampling unit must be connected between the mask or mouthpiece and the two-way valve.) While all of the standard CPET measurements are acquired in tests done in this arrangement with supplemental oxygen, it is important to be aware that significant errors can arise from the oxygen uptake measurements, despite appropriate pretest calibration. If room air is drawn in from a mask leak, the system calculated oxygen consumption will be inappropriately high, and the respiratory R inappropriately low. However the primary goal for the CPET in this setting is to identify the maximal ergometer watt level the patient can reach and to exclude exercise cardiac abnormalities, so this does not invalidate use of the CPET. The CO_2 production measurement is not influenced by mask leak, so the $\dot{V}CO_2$ will provide a reasonable estimate of the $\dot{V}O_2$, especially because severe COPD patients are unable to develop the normal hyperventilation seen with maximal exercise in subjects without lung disease.

With or without oxygen supplementation, a common approach to the aerobic training of COPD patients within a pulmonary rehabilitation program is to exercise the patient at 75% of the maximal ergometer watt setting or the treadmill speed and grade reached at 75% of the total treadmill exercise time. Because patients with severe COPD have very poor cardiovascular fitness by virtue of their enforced sedentary existence, the initial duration of exercise may be 15 minutes or less, but with a goal of extending exercise time to 45 minutes. Similar to the cardiovascular rehab programs, a standard approach is to exercise patients at least three times a week for six to eight weeks.

TRAINING-ASSOCIATED EXERCISE CHANGES IN A PULMONARY REHAB PATIENTS

Successful completion of a pulmonary rehabilitation program is not associated with any change in resting pulmonary function measurements or any increase in maximal oxygen uptake. However, they will consistently demonstrate the capacity to exercise longer at any fixed submaximal exercise level. They also show a lower ventilation requirement and respiratory rate at any given submaximal level, with decreased sense of exercise-associated dyspnea. Measurements of submaximal exercise inspiratory capacity in COPD patients before and after training have demonstrated an increase in exercise inspiratory capacity, suggesting less air trapping, most likely as a result of the reduced respiratory rate.

SUMMARY POINTS

- For patients entering a cardiac rehabilitation program, a standard CPET provides a measurement of maximal exercise heart rate, and from that heart exercise range, can be calculated (HRR = Resting HR − MaxHR). Aerobic training can then be initiated with a goal of maintaining training heart rate at a desired fraction of the HRR (ordinarily between 60% and 75% of HRR).
- Cardiac rehab patients who complete 2–3 months in a supervised exercise program show improvement in $\dot{V}O_2$ max and in addition show a ventilatory threshold that takes place later in the exercise effort.
- The benefits from the aerobic exercise portion of a pulmonary rehabilitation come from being able to exercise at a submaximal level for longer periods of time with less subjective dyspnea. There ordinarily is no improvement in maximal oxygen uptake, and no improvements take place in static pulmonary function tests.

20

Workplace exercise

Modern lifestyle and technology have greatly reduced the role of physical labor in the workforce, but there still are many jobs that require prolonged physical work. Examples of these jobs include factory or construction work, logging, carpentry, firefighting, coal and hard-rock mining, crewing in commercial fishing, and landscaping, to name just a few.

The purpose of this chapter is to describe the role of CPET in quantitating and estimating the work capacity of individuals over a range of physical jobs. These evaluations provide important data for estimating the ability of a subject to perform certain jobs as well as determining disabilities incurred on and off the job.

WORKPLACE CONDITIONS

Working a full shift in a physical job requires being able to perform the tasks of the job successfully and safely for the entire time. These jobs entail a mixture of both high and low intensity, the former to perform the task, the latter to recover and plan for the next time of exertion. There can be times of very high exertion above one's level of sustainable work that cannot be endured for long, but most jobs have tasks that require heavy exertion at a level that is intermittently sustainable. Other factors, such as heat, cold, stress, and danger also may influence physical performance and need to be taken into consideration when evaluating the requirements of a job.

EVALUATION OF PHYSICAL REQUIREMENTS

Most jobs do not come with precise descriptions of what levels of strength and endurance are required, but investigators have looked at several methods to derive good estimates of the physical characteristics needed for certain jobs.

Three different approaches include

1. Measurement of $\dot{V}O_2$ with portable devices to determine the energy required to perform higher levels of exertion during the shifts,
2. Continuous measurements of heart rate to determine and quantitate the proportion of time dedicated to various levels of exertion, and
3. Measurement of caloric intake to maintain a constant body weight.

The measurements, especially of $\dot{V}O_2$ and heart rate from CPET, in individuals can give a fairly accurate estimate of what levels of exertion are expended throughout a typical workday. Measurement of $\dot{V}O_2$ even with lightweight portable systems is tedious and does not give a realistic summary of a work shift; whereas, continuous tracking of heart rates is simple and, if correlated with CPET results, can give one insight into the course of the day and quantitate times of high and low exertion. If work conditions are fairly predictable and constant from an environmental perspective and if the same large muscle masses are used, then a CPET can be done on either a treadmill or cycle ergometer. The heart rate can then be correlated with $\dot{V}O_2$ so that acceptable approximations of energy expenditure throughout a shift can be made. This technique is not precise and does not pertain to jobs that do not use similar large muscle groups but still affords the clinician and worker valuable information for work advisement and disability determination.

General guidelines are available for a variety of jobs that provide industries, workers, and clinicians some direction of what an individual can do.

Although some level of aerobic fitness is necessary to perform an eight-hour shift, knowledge of maximal capacity is more important. That information is critical because some jobs occasionally require high levels of exertion for short periods of time, and one needs to be able to estimate energy reserve that subjects can perform. It is also important for reasons of safety so that employers and workers can be assigned to appropriate jobs. Thus, data derived from CPET can be crucial in making appropriate determinations.

ENERGY EXPENDITURE

No one can maintain eight hours of work at an unsustainable level, and there is a great deal of variability between individuals on their level of endurance and ability to perform occasional high levels of exertion. These capabilities will change with age and vary in environmental conditions. It is thought that a worker can carry out repeated levels of work at 30%–40% of maximal capability during an eight-hour day. Jobs can then be classified from light to extremely heavy, based on actual measurements of $\dot{V}O_2$ or heart rate.

For instance, coastal fisherman are estimated to exert themselves over a full day at 34%–39% of their maximal aerobic capacity while undergoing occasional high levels of exertion up to 80% of peak capacity. Being able to perform at such a high level is unavoidable when a task needs to be performed. Similar patterns are seen in lumberjacks, whereas manual laborers who can set their own pace without moments of high exertion operate at less than 40% of their maximal capacity at a steady pace.

Estimates of energy expenditure and heart rate during a spectrum of intermittent or sustainable levels of work (from Astrand et al. 2003) are listed below:

Workload	Oxygen consumption (L/min)	Heart rate (BPM)
Light	0.5	<90
Moderate	0.5–1.0	90–110
Heavy	1.0–1.5	110–130
Very heavy	1.5–2.0	130–150
Extremely heavy	>2.0	150–170

Energy expenditure for work is paid for by the burning of calories and adding those estimates to the basal metabolic rate, which is usually about 2000 kcal depending on body size. Physical activity for work can add anywhere from 1200–5000 kcal per day. Most jobs that are considered light work expend about 2 kcal/min, whereas some heavy intensity jobs may require 7.5–10 kcal/min.

DETERMINATION OF DISABILITY

Physicians are often asked to make determinations of disability after an injury or illness or occupational environmental exposure. To do so is an imprecise science, but several important factors need to be utilized to come up with some sort of evaluation.

First, a careful history—occupation, medical, family, social—must be taken. That information then puts a work evaluation in perspective and also may reveal environmental exposures that may have an insidious or overt effect on the patient's health and job.

Second, an appropriate physical exam must be done.

Third, focused blood work should be pursued to unveil things like thyroid, adrenal, renal, or hematologic (anemias) abnormalities that could affect physical performance.

Fourth, cardiac and pulmonary evaluations, as needed, may reveal unsuspected abnormalities that could be life-threatening.

Finally, if those data are available, then pulmonary function tests and CPET add invaluable information and will give specific data that can be used to assess a patient's ability to perform various workloads, based on the information of expected capacities for specific work. These evaluations are best made by a clinician who is familiar with CPET and work expectations.

This sort of workup is valuable for someone entertaining certain types of work, as well as workers who have been performing work satisfactorily who then become ill or injured. Patient safety and fairness to the patient is paramount.

REFERENCE

Astrand P-O, Rodahl K, Dahl HA, Stromme SB. 2003. *Textbook of Work Physiology* (4th Edition), Human Kinetics Publisher, Champaign, IL USA.

21

Exercise at altitude

Both acute and chronic exposure to high altitude produce well-defined effects on physical performance. Persons travelling to altitude for work or recreation may first note altitude-related exercise symptoms around 1300 meters (or 4200 feet) and those symptoms increase progressively at higher elevations. As one ascends to higher altitudes, the fraction of oxygen in ambient air remains the same at 0.2093, whereas the barometric pressure decreases resulting in a lower oxygen content for a fixed volume of air. Thus, with ascent, the inspired partial pressure of oxygen as it enters the airways drops from the sea-level value of 150 mmHg to 130 mmHg at 1300 meters to 105 mm Hg at 3000 meters (9700 feet). Both acute and chronic adaptations take place during sojourns to altitude that help reduce the effects of the lower oxygen availability in the inspired air. These adaptations take place in all of the organ systems involved with the transport and utilization of oxygen by exercising muscle. The immediate and longer term responses to altitude acclimatization are discussed by organ system in this chapter. Finally, the effects on exercise performance and the benefits of athletic training at altitude are discussed, taking the known effects of acclimatization into account.

- Ventilation—immediate and ongoing
- Cardiovascular—immediate and ongoing
- Blood—days to weeks and ongoing
- Tissue—weeks to months
- Exercise performance
- Training at altitude

VENTILATION

Upon acute exposure to high altitude, alveolar ventilation is increased as hypoxemia stimulates the peripheral chemosensors in the carotid bodies. While the response is immediate, with ongoing altitude exposure over weeks or longer, there is a further increase in resting and exercise ventilation, producing a yet lower alveolar PCO_2 and higher alveolar PO_2 (Figure 21.1). This ongoing adaptation is important for patients, sojourners, and athletes and results in a higher arterial content of oxygen. There is variability among individuals with the extent of this ventilation acclimatization that may affect susceptibility to altitude illnesses, tolerance to living at higher altitudes, and tolerance for patients with underlying heart and lung disease.

Furthermore, it is important to realize that ambient hypoxia and subsequent hypoxemia stimulates alveolar ventilation such that the ventilator equivalent at rest and during exercise will be increased. This increase should be accounted for during any CPET at high altitude. The work of breathing for any altitude will be greater for any given workload or energy output and can be a major factor that limits exercise at very high altitudes (Figure 21.2).

CARDIOVASCULAR

The cardiac response to high altitude exposure reflects the body's initial and subsequent adaptations to optimize oxygen delivery and is influenced by the course and rate of adaptation by the other organ systems. Upon acute exposure to high altitude, there is an increase in cardiac output both at rest and at fixed levels of exercise compared with low altitude. The increase in cardiac output is achieved primarily by an increase in heart rate. This response has been documented in subjects exposed to altitudes as high as 4000 meters during the first two to four weeks, but after that period

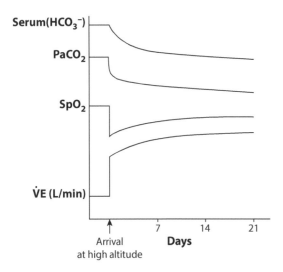

Figure 21.1 Ventilatory acclimatization over time showing progressive increase in ventilation, increase in oxygen saturation (SpO_2), concurrent respiratory alkalosis, and later compensatory metabolic acidosis reflected in a decrease in serum bicarbonate.

of time as other adaptive responses occur, cardiac output re-equilibrates to sea level values. As acclimatization occurs, cardiac output in relation to work level is the same as low altitude.

The initial increase in heart rate is most likely mediated by hypoxia-induced catecholamines. With acute exposure or simulated hypoxia up to 4000 meters, resting heart rate may be 50%–60% above sea level, rates that, with acclimatization, should return close to sea-level values. Exercise

heart rates will follow a similar pattern. The heart rate at peak exercise is reduced at altitude, which may merely reflect the overall decrease in $\dot{V}O_2$ max. For instance, at extreme altitude (equivalent to the summit of Mt Everest), the maximum heart rate is about 115 bpm, but the $\dot{V}O_2$ max in these subjects is only 1 L/min, whereas at sea level, their $\dot{V}O_2$ max was 5 L/min (Figure 21.3).

Stroke volume is decreased at rest and during exercise in both acclimatized individuals and high-altitude natives. At moderate to extreme altitudes, cardiac contractility is maintained in spite of decreased cardiac volumes, myocardial hypoxia, and pulmonary hypertension from hypoxic pulmonary vasoconstriction. Prolonged exposure to extreme altitude (>8000 meters), however, leads to an 11% decrease in myocardial mass and an 18% decrease in cardiac energetics measured by PCr/ATP ratios, findings not dissimilar to patients with cardiac ischemia, presumably secondary to myocardial hypoxia.

On ascent to altitude, systemic blood pressure (SBP), both at rest and during exercise, rises, most likely secondary to a rise in catecholamines. However, over ten days to three weeks, SBP returns to sea-level values. Furthermore, in many high-altitude native populations, SBP has a much lower prevalence than in lowlanders.

Breathing hypoxic air produces an immediate increase in pulmonary artery pressure. The origin of this response may be a vestigial reflex from birth when such a response is necessary to make the immediate transition from placental

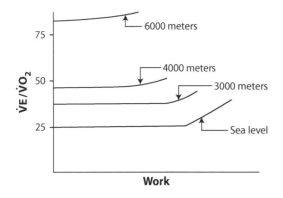

Figure 21.2 Ventilatory equivalent ($\dot{V}E/\dot{V}O_2$) during exercise at sea level and representative altitudes showing the progressive increase in ventilation ($\dot{V}E$) at comparable workloads.

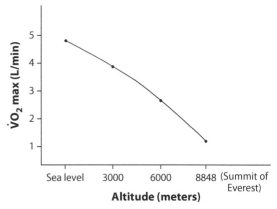

Figure 21.3 Decrease in $\dot{V}O_2$ max with ascent to high altitude.

to pulmonary gas exchange. Hypoxic pulmonary vasoconstriction (HPVR) and pulmonary hypertension (PHTN) develop in all individuals upon ascent and while living at high altitude. This response exhibits a wide degree of variability between individuals, and that variability may be critically relevant to functional performance and predisposition to high-altitude pulmonary edema. PHTN increases with exercise at high altitude to a much greater extent than observed at sea level and may impair right ventricular output and thus overall cardiac output. This supposition is supported by studies demonstrating that administration of pulmonary vasodilators such as endothelin-1 (ET-1) blockers result in a partial attenuation of the HPVR response to hypoxia and improvement in exercise performance. Thus, it is important for clinicians who evaluate patients for travel to high altitude to be aware that that the presence of PHTN at sea level represents a substantial risk for cor pulmonale upon ascent to altitude and that exercise at altitude will be poorly tolerated.

BLOOD

The hematologic response to high-altitude exposure develops over time and has both positive and negative effects on oxygen delivery. The hematologic response to hypoxia is triggered by the gene transcription factor hypoxia-inducible-factor-1-alpha (HIF-1-alpha), initiating a cascade of downstream genes including those for the red-blood-cell growth-factor erythropoietin (EPO). Upon acute exposure to hypoxia, EPO increases within the first couple of hours, but it takes 10–14 days for appreciable increases in hemoglobin and oxygen delivery to become apparent. EPO then decreases when the body's need for increased oxygen delivery decreases in conjunction with other adaptive mechanisms.

It is not clear what the optimal level of hemoglobin (Hgb) response to chronic hypoxia might be, but levels above 18 gm/dL result in increased blood viscosity, impaired microvascular perfusion, and thus impaired oxygen delivery to the cells and mitochondria. It is important for the clinician evaluating a patient or athlete to be aware of this hematologic adaptation effect of high altitude and to be aware of the hemoglobin level whether it is high, low, or normal for that altitude. With polycythemia, O_2 delivery is not

only impaired, but the increased viscosity leads to increased pulmonary vascular resistance and PHTN.

PERIPHERAL ADAPTATIONS

There is still controversy about the adaptations taking place in the peripheral tissues with exposure and habitation at high altitude. Ideally, as the supply of oxygen decreases, both capillary and mitochondrial density should increase, such as has been documented in aerobic training at low altitude. These morphologic changes result in greater oxygen supply (capillary density) and decreased diffusion distance to the mitochondria in an environment where the driving pressures for oxygen are lower. At moderate altitudes ($\sim$<3000 m), this adaptation may in fact occur.

With prolonged exposure to very high altitudes (>6000 m), the utilization of oxygen is achieved by a different strategy that may be a function of the decreased activity at altitude, as opposed to the stimulus per se of tissue hypoxia. A decrease in diffusion distance and a practical increase in the capillary/cell density is achieved by a decrease in the muscle-fiber size. Mitochondrial density also appears to decrease.

EXERCISE PERFORMANCE

In spite of the aforementioned adaptations that decrease the loss of both endurance and maximum exercise performance at altitude, there is not full recouping of sea-level capacity. This fact is important for both athletes and patients with cardiopulmonary disease living and/or traveling to high altitude. A study 50 years ago, prior to the 1968 Olympics in Mexico City (approximately 2200 meters), showed an average drop in $\dot{V}O_2$ max of 16% (range 9%–22%) upon acute exposure to 2300 meters. Nineteen days of acclimatization at that altitude resulted in less of a drop (average 11%, range 6%–16%)—improvement but not full recovery at that modest altitude.

Many studies at extreme altitudes, including both field and hypobaric chamber studies to the equivalent of the summit of Mt Everest, have shown a predictable decrease in maximum oxygen consumption. For instance, the $\dot{V}O_2$ max after prolonged exposure to very high altitudes ($\sim$>6000 m) was 20% of what it was at sea level—some work (one L O_2/min vs. 5 L O_2/min), but not a lot and certainly not sustainable.

With these predictable diminutions of aerobic capacity at known altitudes, the use of CPET to document the progress, up and down, of performance is quite helpful in athletes who are living or training at altitude (see next section.)

There have been a number of clinical studies to evaluate the effect of altitude on patients with COPD, pulmonary hypertension, coronary artery disease, and dysrhythmias. The purpose has been to formulate safety guidelines both for patients living at or travelling to high altitude, as well as patients with pulmonary disease travelling in commercial airliners, where the cabin pressure simulates ascent to about 2100–2400 meters. Because of the immediate and sustained increase in pulmonary artery pressure on altitude exposure, patients with known pulmonary hypertension should not sojourn to high altitude. CPET testing can be helpful for certain patients in which a full evaluation, above and beyond looking for a drop in oxygen saturation, may be helpful in advising a patient going for recreation or to live in the highlands.

TRAINING AT HIGH ALTITUDE FOR ATHLETIC PERFORMANCE

In the 1968 Olympics held at 2300 meters in Mexico City, the Kenyan-runner Kip Keino defeated the favored American runner, Jim Ryun. Keino had grown up at a similar altitude in Kenya. People assumed that his living and training at high altitude was the key to his success so much so that many runners from all over the world started moving to locations that simulated 2300 meters. The other unconsidered factor might be that Keino had run many miles to school for many years!

Subsequently, a number of studies looked into the effect of various long-term altitude exposures on aerobic performance. A number of variables were measured including race times, but the most important data, maximum aerobic capacity ($\dot{V}O_2$ max) and lactate threshold (LT), emanated from classic CPET testing.

Investigators looked at the effect on training by living and training at low altitude (LLTL), living and training at altitude (LHTH), living low and training high (LLTH), and living high and training low (LHTL). With a few caveats, most studies have shown that LHTL provides the most benefit, thought to be secondary to the positive effects of the hypoxic stimulus while allowing a higher intensity of training and recovery at lower altitude. To choose the optimal altitude that is not too high or too low, studies have shown that 2000–2450 meters is optimal, whereas, 2800 meters appears to be too high.

The single factor that best explained the benefit was an increase in red blood cell mass, although this response was somewhat variable among subjects, even in studies that insured adequate iron stores for the erythropoietic response. To attain an optimal response, it is recommended that athletes stay at altitude for at least three to four weeks and maintain 16–22 hours of hypoxic exposure per day.

Because of the difficulty of gaining a high-altitude training location (expense, having to move, etc.) some athletes have accessed "hypoxic tents" that can be placed over their beds and adjusted to various altitudes. The success of this technique has not been confirmed in large part because it is felt that the normal sleep cycle per day is not long enough to invoke or sustain some of the beneficial effects such as erythropoiesis and ventilatory acclimatization.

If one is undergoing altitude training for competition at low altitude, then one question is: how long do the positive effects last? The increase in red blood cell mass has significant decay by 14 days, and ventilatory decay is more rapid, although not well studied. Thus, it seems prudent to compete within two to three days after descent.

If athletes choose to go to these extraordinary measures, testing the outcomes is critical so that one does not undertake unnecessary and excessive steps that may not help for an individual athlete. Thus, the most detailed analysis of improvement or decline comes from CPET testing and simple blood work (CBC and iron studies). The most important outcome variables are $\dot{V}O_2$ max, $\dot{V}E$, $\dot{V}E/\dot{V}O_2$, and measurements of sustainable work (changes in lactate or ventilatory thresholds). CPET testing at low altitude and blood work should be undertaken before and at regular intervals, starting at about one month. If no beneficial effects are detected for the individual, then one must question the effort.

SUMMARY

This chapter has briefly reviewed the natural process of acclimatization to high altitude and the effect of the hypoxic environment on exercise performance and has supplemented the chapter on training by looking at the pros and cons of including exposure to an hypoxic environment. It also emphasizes the importance of CPET testing on determining the beneficial and potentially deleterious effects of exposure to high altitude in both patients and competitive athletes.

22

Exercise in heat and cold

The principles of human thermoregulation do not ordinarily play a significant role in the conduct or interpretation of laboratory CPET testing. However, understanding the effect of environmental temperature on exercise responses is important for counseling patients who will be exercising in challenging environments.

This chapter describes heat generation by the exercising muscles, the potential effect of this heat generation on work output, and the body's exercise adaptations to the climatic extremes of cold and heat.

PHYSIOLOGIC RESPONSE TO THE HEAT OF EXERCISE

There is a narrow range of ambient temperature (28°C–30°C) for an unclothed resting human to maintain homeostasis and survive. The thermal gradient between the body and ambient air dictates the strategy that the body employs to remain relatively euthermic. At rest, the adult body consumes 200–300 mL O_2/minute for fuel metabolism, producing 60–90 kcal of heat per hour. That heat is dissipated by direct radiation to the environment, convection of surface heat by wind, conduction of heat from the body's surface to another surface, and evaporation of water from the skin and respiratory tract.

Muscular exercise proportionately increases both metabolic rate and overall heat production. Exercising muscle is a chemical engine, and like all engines, consuming its fuel produces both work and heat. A subject generating 100 watts of power while pedaling a cycle ergometer will also generate well over 200 watts of heat. Hence, for a fit subject capable of heavy sustained exercise, body temperature rises even during a routine CPET by 38–39°C. (Note that this extent of exercise-associated hyperthermia not an issue for patients with significant exercise impairment, as they can generate only a far lower maximal watt output.) For the very fit subjects giving a maximal effort, core temperature does not continue to rise further because of enhanced loss of heat by sweating and evaporation. The rise in core temperature during exercise triggers a reflex resulting in both peripheral vasodilatation and activation of the sweat glands for cooling by evaporation. The increase in blood flow to the skin during exercise represents about five percent of the cardiac output but can rise to 20% with sustained exercise in very warm environments (see Chapter 14 for discussion of modest differences in gender). This "cardiac steal" robs oxygen delivery from the muscles of locomotion and limits the maximal oxygen uptake, as very little oxygen is extracted from blood flowing to the skin. Thus sustained exercise at a fixed power output in a hot environment produces no change in oxygen consumption, but requires a higher cardiac output and heart rate. However this diversion of blood flow to skin during exercise in hot environments is essential to prevent an unregulated rise in core temperature and the associated severe central nervous system complications of hyperthermia.

PRINCIPLES OF HEAT TRANSFER

There are four mechanisms of thermal transfer resulting in a gain or loss of body heat:

1. Radiant heat loss without a transfer medium. This is the most common cause of clinical hypothermia in patients who have been injured in their homes, lying in a still environment for one or more days.

2. Conduction of heat from one surface to another. An example of loss of body heat by conduction is a person lying on a cold surface or in water.
3. Convection from air blowing past the body, e.g., the wind chill factor. Moving water can also "wick" heat away from a body, a combination of conduction and convection.
4. Evaporation of water on the skin, ordinarily from active sweating. This is the most important mechanism to decrease the accumulation of body heat during exercise in hot environments.

ADAPTATION TO HEAT AND COLD

Over many millennia, humans have progressively developed improvements in shelter and clothing to maintain a euthermic environment in which survival and performance are maintained. In addition, however, when people live or athletes train in consistently hot or cold environments, individual physiologic acclimatization occurs that improves functionality in that environment.

HEAT

Over a few days of exposure to a hot environment, the sweating response is increased, resulting in more effective core temperature control with exertion. The body utilizes evaporation as the most important strategy to minimize the rise in core temperature during exercise, and this response is augmented over time by prolonged exposure to heat, while the amount of heat lost by radiation and convection remains constant. If a subject is exercising with wind or water flowing over the body, there is an additional loss of heat by convection.

The sweating adaptation to sustained heat exposure is preceded, however, by the immediate increase in blood flow to the skin, producing the above-described diversion of blood flow away from muscles during heavy exercise. After seven to ten days of continued exposure to the heat, there is an increase in plasma volume to partially compensate for the newly expanded blood flow to the largest organ system, the skin, and thus improve blood flow to muscle during exercise. Cardiodynamic responses at rest return toward normal, with an increase in stroke volume and decrease in resting heart rate. It is not totally clear that this adaptation is augmented with regular exercise in the cold.

From a practical standpoint for work or athletic performance, these concepts of heat acclimatization are important to understand because several days of exposure to a hot environment are critical for any planned bout of sustained heavy exercise in that environment.

COLD

The first response of an unclothed human to exposure to a cold environment is to shiver. Shivering occurs from stimulation of peripheral cold receptors and occurs with normal core temperatures. Heavy shivering at rest can increase the metabolic rate up to five times the resting value and thus increase heat production, maintaining normal body temperatures for at least a couple of hours. (Obviously, the same level of heat production can be achieved by moderate exercise.) If body temperature drops after time, shivering will continue until a core temperature of about 33.3°C, at which point shivering stops. The reason for the loss of this response with increasing hypothermia is not clear.

Cold adaptation over time results in a decrease of the shivering response, and this adaptation can occur both with prolonged exposure as well as intermittent daily exposures of 30–60 minutes to cold. It can also occur over seasons, for instance in individuals whose occupation, such as seafood divers, find themselves exposed to cold water for several months. The acclimatization response of decreased shivering is lost in the "off-season." Athletes in certain winter sport competitions also may benefit from pre-acclimatization.

In cold, but not extreme cold environments, the energy/work ratio remains constant, but peripheral thermosensors note a decrease in skin temperature and stimulate vasoconstriction of cutaneous blood flow. This response results in a decreased but not ablated sweating response, decreases skin temperature and thus heat loss by radiation, and subsequently maintains core temperature.

THERMAL MALADIES

The discussion of maladies incurred from the heat and cold is not in the purview of this text on applications for CPET, but it is important to know that exposure and exercise in hot and cold environments can result in a variety of illnesses, most transient while some of them result in long-lasting effects or death. It is difficult to erase the image of the Swiss woman Olympic marathon runner staggering and ataxic into the Los Angeles stadium in 1984 with severe hyperthermia.

In the cold, one can incur mild, moderate, or severe hypothermia and a number of metabolic and peripheral injuries such as dehydration, coagulopathies, and frostbite; in the heat, the recognized illnesses are dehydration, heat exhaustion, and heat stroke. The last entity can be fatal and may be associated with severe coagulopathies, circulatory collapse, and anhidrosis.

Clinicians doing CPET testing may receive consults in their laboratories to test patients and athletes who have suffered mild to severe heat illnesses; and although there are no exercise responses specifically associated with heat intolerance, it is critical to make sure that their exercise performance is normal, as significant reductions in exercise capacity with cardiac limitation are associated with predisposition to thermal illnesses.

SUMMARY POINTS

Although the clinician doing CPET consultations will rarely incur the direct effects of changes in ambient temperatures, this chapter described the following issues:

1. The body's normal metabolic response to exercise includes the production of heat that is proportional to the level of work sustained.
2. The principles of heat transfer to and from the human body explain the adaptations to the onset and continuation of exercise.
3. The influence of environmental fluctuations of temperature on physiologic responses and exercise performance.
4. The body's ability to achieve long-term adaptations to either a hot or cold environment, a topic important both to workers and athletes.
5. A brief listing of illnesses often confronted in cold or hot environments.

Index

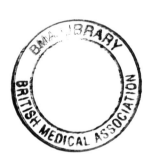